IMMUNOLOGY

Immunology

William Anderson, Ph.D.

Professor of Biochemistry

Department of Biochemistry

University of New Mexico School of Medicine

Albuquerque, New Mexico

**Fence Creek
Publishing**

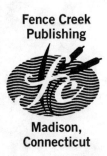

**Madison,
Connecticut**

Typesetter: Pagesetters, Brattleboro, VT
Printer: Port City Press, Baltimore, MD
Illustrations by Oxford Designers and Illustrators, Oxford, England
Distributors:

United States and Canada
Blackwell Science, Inc.
Commerce Place
350 Main Street
Malden, MA 02148
Telephone orders: 800-215-1000 or 781-388-8250
Fax orders: 781-388-8270

Australia
Blackwell Science, PTY LTD.
54 University Street
Carlton, Victoria 3053
Telephone orders: 61-39-347-0300
Fax orders: 61-39-347-5001

Outside North America and Australia
Blackwell Science, LTD.
c/o Marston Book Service, LTD.
P.O. Box 269
Abingdon Oxon, OX 14 4XN England
Telephone orders: 44-1-235-465500
Fax orders: 44-1-235-465555

1 2 3 4 5 6 7 8 9 10

CONTENTS

PREFACE

Our understanding of the immune system is changing. The system has been viewed solely as a method of defense against foreign organisms. More recently, however, the view has begun to shift towards that expressed by Tomio Tada (*Annual Reviews of Immunology*, 1997), who sees the immune system as an independent regulatory system, or supersystem, that essentially defines its own fate and actions. This changing view along with the current proliferation of knowledge about the immune response has created an environment of exciting challenges in which teachers help students learn about and appreciate this dynamic system.

Traditionally, students of immunology followed the development of specific topics by assimilating the experimental findings that led to our understanding of a concept and then moved on to the next concept. While this approach can be fascinating, rich in history, and can develop an appreciation of all aspects of the immune system, including an experimental approach to the subject, it does not address the learning styles of all students. Moreover, for those students not involved in an intensive course of training in immunology, such as first-year medical students, the amount of material can be daunting. I have watched many students try to learn immunology by memorizing its lexicon without gaining an understanding of how the system referred to by those words functions.

A new and sometimes confounding factor in the medical school environment is the increased application of problem-based learning, which has significantly curtailed the time given to formal lectures and has appropriately placed more of the responsibility for learning on the students. But this change places another constraint on educators more familiar with traditional methods of immunology education.

This book is organized in two parts. Part I, The Basics, attempts to help students construct their own framework for understanding the immune system. The clinical cases provide examples of what happens during an immune response and why and emphasize the relationship between the immune system and other organ systems. Part II, Learning Issues, presents a collection of focused issues that has evolved from students' difficulties in understanding the immune response. The issues build on Part I, using more detail and vocabulary, and reinforcing the basic concepts. This is an iterative process of immunology education. The material is repeated when the student goes to reference books, reviews, or primary sources, and when his or her knowledge of the immune system is called on to solve a clinical problem.

There are several outstanding immunology textbooks on the market, and this book is not designed to replace any of them. Rather, it is designed to help students organize and understand the very basic principles of the immune response. This book should provide the fundamental concepts to help students craft questions which can be answered by other textbooks, reference books, review articles, and original research reports. It is meant to be the beginning of a journey into lifelong learning about the immune system and its role in normal and abnormal physiology rather than the sole source of information about immunology.

This approach has grown out of more than two decades of teaching immunology to undergraduate students. It was shaped, in large part, by students' questions and comments and by listening to their struggles to learn immunology; it was also shaped by the constraints of the new, integrated approaches to medical education. When asked to write this book, the charge was to provide an introduction to the basic principles of immunology for first-year medical students, an introduction that does not depend on memorizing the entire lexicon of the discipline but allows the acquisition of language to grow as the student delves deeper into his or her study of the immune system. The goal of this book is to help the student build his or her own framework for understanding the immune system's biologic role. This understanding can then expand as the student's experience and understanding of immunopathology expands.

William Anderson, Ph.D.

ACKNOWLEDGMENTS

I am indebted to several outstanding colleagues in the areas of immunology and education for support and discussion while writing this book. Professor Sei Tokuda and my wife, Rochelle, deserve special acknowledgment. I am most indebted, however, to my students, who over the last 20 years have been willing to share their struggles with learning immunology.

INTRODUCTION

Immunology is one of ten titles in the *Integrated Medical Sciences (IMS) Series* from Fence Creek Publishing. These books have been designed as course supplements and aids for board review for first- and second-year medical students. Rather than focusing on the individual basic science disciplines, the books in the *IMS Series* have been designed to highlight the points of integration between the sciences, including clinical correlations where appropriate. Each chapter begins with a clinical case, the resolution of which requires the application of basic science concepts to clinical problems. Extensive use of margin notes, figures, tables, and questions illuminates core biomedical concepts with which medical students often have difficulty.

Each book in the *IMS Series* shares common features and formats. Attempts have been made to present difficult concepts in a brief and focused format and to provide a pedagogical aid that facilitates both knowledge acquisition and also review.

Given the long gestation period necessary to publish a book, it is often impossible for publishers to keep pace with the changes and advances that occur so rapidly. However, the authors and the publishers recognize the need to have access to the most current information and are committed to keeping *Immunology* as up-to-date as possible between editions. As the field of immunology evolves, updates to this text may be posted on our web site periodically at http://www.fencecreek.com.

We hope that the student finds the format and the text material relevant, interesting, and challenging. The authors, as well as the Fence Creek staff, welcome your comments and suggestions for use in future editions.

PART I: THE BASICS

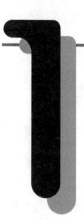

BIOLOGIC ROLE OF THE IMMUNE SYSTEM

CHAPTER OUTLINE

INTRODUCTION OF CLINICAL CASE

Jill Smythe, a 12-year-old girl, was brought to her primary care physician by her parents, because they were worried about her recent weight loss and fatigue. Her parents were really puzzled by the weight loss because, they said, "she is hungry all of the time but is continually eating and drinking." Her urinary frequency was also considerably increased. Urinalysis showed the presence of glucose. The level of glucose in the blood was also significantly increased.

BRIEF HISTORY OF IMMUNOLOGY

Our current understanding of the immune system is based on the collected observations and experiments of numerous individuals that extend far beyond the scope of this book. Consequently, only a cursory review can be attempted here.

Two characteristics of the immune system were recognized very early and were repeatedly commented on in writings about protection against infectious disease. The first characteristic is the unique

> **Characteristics of the Acquired Immune Response:**
> • *Memory*
> • *Specificity*

specificity of immunologic reactions. The specificity of the immune response is of such precision that it can select one cell among many or it can identify one isomer of a compound and react with only these selected components and not the adjacent cells or the other isomer. The second characteristic of the immune system is its ability to remember previous encounters and respond more rapidly and vigorously on second exposure. Depending on the nature of the antigen and the type of immune response generated, this immunologic memory can be either of short or long duration. For example, the current recommendation for tetanus immunization boosters is that they be given every decade, while single immunizations are recommended for other infections, because they provide permanent immunity.

Probably the earliest report of an immune response dates back to early Egyptian records, in which a term roughly analogous to inflammation is used to describe the death of the Pharaoh following a bee sting. However, more commonly cited as the first description of immunity is the historian Thucydides' discussion of plague, in which he wrote: "It was with those who had recovered from the disease that the sick and the dying found most compassion. These knew what it was from experience, and had now no fear for themselves; for the same man was never attacked twice." This observation opened an era in which many theories were proposed to explain the mechanisms behind the observation of acquired immunity: Did the first encounter with the infectious agent expel or deplete bad humors in the individual? Did the first exposure to an infectious agent consume some component that was essential for the growth of the infectious organism? These were but two of the earliest theories to explain the remarkable observations of immunologic memory and specificity.

At the end of the 19th century, the practices of immunization and the questions asked about the immune system opened a truly incredible era of research and discovery. However, the knowledge gained during that period is dwarfed by the rate and magnitude of current immunologic advances. This rapid accumulation of knowledge and changing understanding of the immune system provide an exciting future and a challenge to the health care provider.

WHAT THE IMMUNE SYSTEM DOES

Protection against Infectious Agents

The brief discussion above and the focus of much of early research concentrated on the role of the immune system in response to foreign substances and protection against infectious disease. Clearly, protection against infectious agents is one major function of the immune system.

Immunologic Surveillance

Jill's current condition presents a major problem in understanding what the immune system does. In her case, components of the immune system initiated a reaction directed against one specific cell type, eliminating those cells and the function they perform. To complicate further our understanding of immunology, it appears that individuals who are not suffering from Jill's autoimmune disease possess identical autoreactive components. In contrast to Jill, their autoimmune response is controlled and a part of normal physiology. In Jill's case, the immune system "decided" to reject a normal tissue, whereas in the normal individual, the immune system, although capable of responding, tolerates the presence of the identical tissue. Jill's condition, then, identifies another role of the immune system—the routine surveillance of all tissues. The immune system is responsible for deciding what tissues may remain and what tissues should be rejected. It routinely surveys all tissues, evaluating cells and cell products, along with components of the extracellular fluid compartment, to remove dead, dying, mutated, altered, or infected components. In this context, autoimmune *reactivity* is common, and it is a necessary component of tissue turnover. Autoimmune *disease*, on the other hand, is less frequent and is an example of altered regulation of a normal response. As knowledge of the immune system expanded, the number of recognized autoimmune conditions grew to such an extent that, depending on which author one reads, autoimmune reactions are responsible for pathology in 10%–50% of the population.

In its surveillance capacity, then, the immune system is unique among organ systems. It continually regenerates itself from a single precursor cell, generating its own diversity and, essentially under its own control, deciding whether to tolerate or reject a tissue or infectious agent. Having decided, it then infiltrates all the tissues and organs of the body, continually surveying the compounds and cells that are present and materials that are being produced by each cell. If the immune system decides that a tissue belongs, then that tissue is tolerated and allowed to remain. If, on the other hand, the cells or molecules are foreign, dying, or simply not tolerated, the immune system coordinates their removal. In Jill's case, her immune system "decided" for unknown reasons that the critical beta cells of the pancreatic islets did not belong, and they were removed. The immune system then is one that takes on the characteristics of what has been described as a supersystem.

HOW THE IMMUNE SYSTEM FUNCTIONS

Activation of the Immune Response

In learning about the immune system, one can define several steps, or processes that occur during the response to any agent. First, the immune system must specifically recognize the agent. Since the immune system is also given the challenge of surveying the products being made by all the cells of the body, it must include mechanisms for evaluating synthetic events taking place inside each nucleated cell. This problem of evaluation is addressed by requiring that each nucleated cell displays all synthetic products on its cell surface for inspection by the immune system. To accomplish these recognition tasks, the immune system needs to generate cells with receptors for any possible structure. This recognition component of the immune system is comprised of the B and T lymphocytes. Fig. 1-1 outlines the cells responsible for the antigen-specific activation of the immune response. The B lymphocytes react to soluble materials, while the sets of T lymphocytes react with antigens presented on the cell surface. In order for the immune system to be activated, both B and T cells must be selected.

Immune Effector Functions

A second function of the immune system is the recruitment of accessory cells to the site where an infectious agent has been detected. Whereas the B and T lymphocytes possess the unique ability to recognize a target, the immune system often depends on and recruits a variety of phagocytic cells, cells with potent cytotoxic activity, to carry out the cytotoxicity and removal of the specific targets identified by the immune system. A summary of the immune system's effector functions is illustrated in Fig. 1-2.

Communication

Finally, the immune system needs to coordinate not only the responses of immunocompetent cells and accessory inflammatory cells, but it must also coordinate inflammatory responses observed in all of the other tissues. This coordination is under the control of soluble autocrine, paracrine, and endocrine factors called cytokines. To understand the immune system, each element of the immune response needs to be understood in more detail.

Five events in the immune response:
- Recognition of specific antigen
- Recruitment of inflammatory cells
- Removal of antigen
- Remembering the immune response
- Repairing tissue damaged by the immune response

RESOLUTION OF CLINICAL CASE

During development, unknown events in Jill's genetic make-up altered the way her immune system interacted with an environmental agent. The events led her system to view specific markers (antigens) on beta cells in the pancreatic islets as foreign. Once this occurred, the stimulated immune system recruited the cells necessary to eliminate the specific target tissue. This process required the coordination both of B cells and different populations of T cells to orchestrate the tissue rejection. In Jill's case, her immune system was able to remove selectively only the insulin-producing beta cells of the pancreas, while leaving intact other pancreatic cells capable of synthesizing glucagon and producing bicarbonate and the digestive enzymes. A component of Jill's

FIGURE 1-1 ▶

Activation of the Immune Response. The immune response is activated when antigen selects (i.e., binds to) one of the antigen-specific lymphocytes of the immune system. One type of antigen-specific cell is the B lymphocyte, which is able to bind directly to the stimulating antigen via a cell-surface antigen receptor. After the B lymphocyte binds the antigen, it eventually develops into a plasma cell, which secretes a soluble antibody molecule containing the identical binding site for antigen that was on the original B lymphocyte. B lymphocytes give rise to humoral immunity or antibody-mediated immunity. A second type of antigen-specific cell is the cytotoxic T cell, also called a CD8 cell. This cell is selected by antigen that is being synthesized in a host cell. The synthesized antigen is chemically changed so that it can be displayed on the cell surface for evaluation by the immune system. CD8 cells give rise to cell-mediated cytotoxicity, which is a component of cell-mediated immunity. The third type of antigen-specific cell, the helper T lymphocyte, or CD4 cell, is selected by a special class of cells called antigen-presenting cells (APCs). The APCs take up soluble materials from the environment and display them on their surface for analysis by the CD4 cells of the immune system. The CD4 class of lymphocyte is complex, in that CD4 cells have two functions: (1) They help both B lymphocytes and CD8 T lymphocytes, and, (2) they mediate a type of local inflammatory reaction called delayed-type hypersensitivity. Both activities depend on communication among the lymphocytes, which is mediated through soluble cellular regulatory products, called cytokines. These important cytokines include, but are not limited to, the interleukins: IL-1, IL-2, IL-4, IL-5, and IL-6.

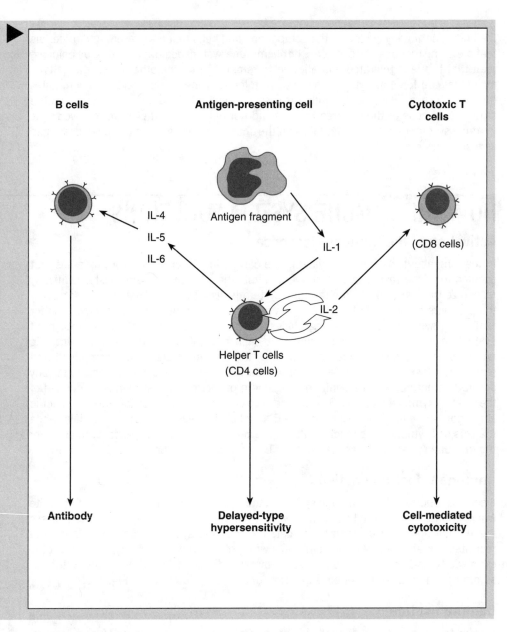

response to the pancreatic cells is the establishment of a memory of the initial encounter. Should the rejected cell type appear again (e.g., a transplant), a much more efficient and rapid removal of the cells would occur on second exposure.

In Jill's case, her immune system very efficiently eliminated her specific beta cells and their functional role in insulin production. To accommodate this loss, Jill needs to supply the insulin that her beta cells once produced.

Jill's autoimmune response demonstrates that the immune system must be viewed as involved in far more physiologic processes than simply protecting against invading microorganisms. This is a system that is highly integrated with all of the other organ systems. It evaluates synthetic products of each cell as well as the cell's environment and then makes decisions about whether or not the cell or its product is consistent with normal physiology.

Jill's immune response is evaluated by first looking globally at the cells and tissues of her immune system, how they are activated, how they can respond to and eliminate antigen, and finally how they communicate with the other organ systems. This initial global view is followed by a more in-depth discussions of some of the key concepts of immunology. This, however, is not the complete immunology story, and students should be prepared to extend their study and understanding of Jill's response by using reference texts, reviews, and other available resources.

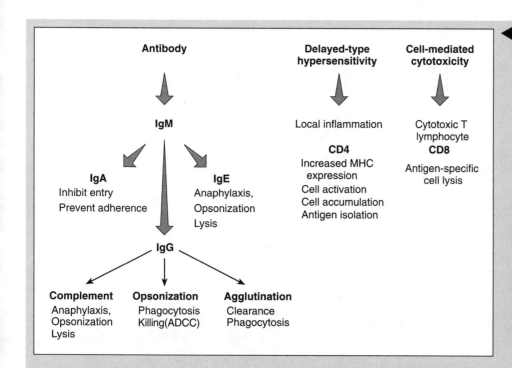

Antibody

↓

IgM

↙   ↓   ↘

IgA   **IgE**
Inhibit entry   Anaphylaxis,
Prevent adherence   Opsonization
                          Lysis

IgG

↙   ↓   ↘

Complement   **Opsonization**   **Agglutination**
Anaphylaxis,   Phagocytosis   Clearance
Opsonization   Killing(ADCC)   Phagocytosis
Lysis

Delayed-type hypersensitivity

↓

Local inflammation

CD4
Increased MHC expression
Cell activation
Cell accumulation
Antigen isolation

Cell-mediated cytotoxicity

↓

Cytotoxic T lymphocyte
CD8

Antigen-specific cell lysis

FIGURE 1-2
Immune Effector Functions. *The immune system has three different methods of eliminating the offending antigen. One method is humoral immunity, which is represented by antibody. There are four different types of antibodies (immunoglobulin): IgM, IgG, IgE, and IgA, and each functions differently in response to antigen. The antibodies interact with other cells and toxic proteins to remove specific antigens (IgM, IgG). Some of the antigen-removal systems include a series of inflammatory proteins called complement; a method to mark foreign materials for phagocytic cells, called opsonization; and the recruitment of antibody-dependent cytotoxic cells (ADCC). Other antibodies (IgA) prevent antigens from adhering to or entering the body, while the IgE antibodies signal inflammatory responses (anaphylaxis). Cell-mediated immunity eliminates antigen either by a direct cellular lysis of target cells, cell-mediated cytotoxicity or by stimulating a local inflammatory response, delayed-type hypersensitivity.*

REFERENCES

Silverstein AM: *A History of Immunology.* San Diego, Academic Press, 1989.
Tada, T: The immune system as a supersystem. *Ann Rev Immunol* 15:1–13, 1997.

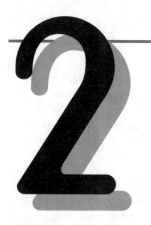

INTRODUCTION TO THE IMMUNE SYSTEM: INNATE AND ACQUIRED IMMUNITY

INTRODUCTION OF CLINICAL CASE

Jimmy Marcus, a 4-year-old boy, was riding his tricycle when he lost control and fell. As a result of his fall, he scraped and injured his hand with a sliver of wood. In addition to the sliver, Jimmy severely twisted his knee. Within a few minutes, both of his injuries began swelling. The injured areas became hot, red, and painful. Moreover, Jimmy could not easily move his knee because of the painful swelling.

> **Hallmarks of an Inflammatory Response**
> *Rubor = Redness*
> *Calor = Heat*
> *Tumor = Swelling*
> *Dolor = Pain*
> *Loss of function*

FUNCTIONS OF THE IMMUNE SYSTEM

Protection against Extracellular Foreign Antigens

One of the most easily understood and most often discussed functions of the immune system is its role in protecting against foreign antigens. Jimmy is an excellent example of this function. Not only is the sliver itself a large foreign object, but the wound it caused provides a route for the introduction of environmental contaminants (e.g., microorganisms, large foreign molecules). In the short time that the sliver has been in Jimmy's hand, his immune system began identifying the spectrum of materials contained on the sliver and initiated mechanisms to remove those agents. In its protective role, the immune system must be prepared to carry out its activities at any entry route of foreign material. This requires the immune system to be mobile and flexible. It must be able to identify foreign antigens rapidly and coordinate a variety of potential host responses. These responses, however, need to differ depending on the route of exposure and the nature of the antigen.

The range of immunologic events that are taking place in response to the foreign antigens in Jimmy's hand are schematically illustrated in Fig. 2-1. A microscopic examination of the wound would show a marked change in the structures of the tissues. The capillaries become more permeable to allow more fluid to enter the tissue. *Phagocytic cells* are entering the area, and by examining the function and metabolism of these cells, it is evident that the cells are activated and rapidly engulfing the foreign materials. In addition to the phagocytes, a system of proteins called *complement* is activated to help Jimmy respond to the introduction of the materials contained on the sliver. Moreover, if Jimmy had previously encountered the materials contained on the sliver, antibody molecules that could bind and aggregate antigens and mark them for removal by the phagocytic cells would already exist or be rapidly produced. In this scenario, Jimmy's response to the sliver identifies one function of the immune system, that of continually surveying the extracellular environment, thereby identifying materials that do not belong and coordinating the activities of phagocytes in the removal of those materials.

Main Functions of Immune System
Continually survey the extracellular space for foreign materials and coordinate their removal.

FIG. 2-1
Summary of Inflammatory Response to Antigen–Antibody Complexes. *Antigen–antibody complexes can activate the complement cascade through the classic pathway. This results in the generation of complement component C3a and other complement anaphylatoxins. These small peptide fragments bind to receptors on tissue mast cells and induce them to release the contents of their preformed granules (degranulation). The granule contents contain histamine and other inflammatory mediators that have potent vasodilation activities and promote the exudation of serum proteins and cells into the inflammatory tissues. Antigen–antibody complexes are also opsonized structures for tissue phagocytes. The resident macrophage rapidly engulfs the opsonized materials and starts producing potent monokines that recruit other inflammatory cells.*

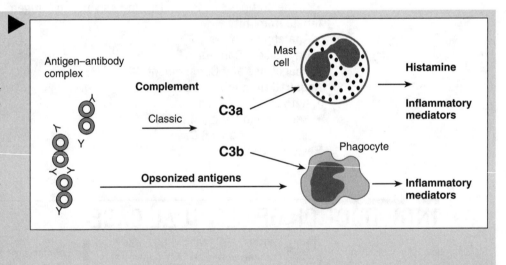

Protection against Intracellular Foreign Antigens

The range of materials that, potentially, could infect Jimmy are not limited only to the organisms that inhabit extracellular fluids. Viruses or bacteria that reside or colonize inside cells could also be contaminating the sliver. To address this additional possibility, the immune system must have the capability of evaluating the intracellular environment for pathogens or for the synthesis of improper or altered self-proteins. The immune system must continually perform this function for all cells having the capability to synthesize macromolecules.

Detecting and Removing Altered Self-Structures

In his tricycle mishap, the sliver was not the only injury sustained by Jimmy. He also twisted his knee and experienced a rapid inflammatory response to the injury, although there was no break in the skin and no introduction of foreign antigen. Fig. 2-2 schematically illustrates the inflammatory events that are happening in Jimmy's knee. Common events are evident in Figs. 2-1 and 2-2. Not only is the immune system responsible for identifying foreign materials, but it must also respond to damaged, dying, or dead tissues. The mechanisms used by the immune system to deal with these different situations are identical; the differences between these responses relate only to the nature of the events that stimulated the immune system.

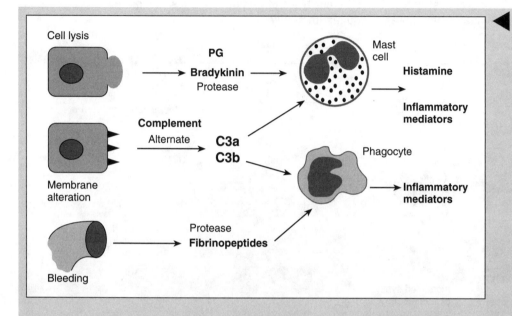

◀ **FIG. 2-2**
Summary of Inflammatory Response to Damaged Tissue. *Physical damage to tissues can lyse cells, alter membrane structures, and cause bleeding into the tissues. Each of these events has the potential to activate the inflammatory response. Cell lysis can activate the kinin cascade, resulting in the formation of bradykinin. Bradykinin is a potent chemical mediator that can increase vascular permeability and vasodilation and cause pain. In addition, the mediator activates arachidonic acid metabolism, resulting in the production of additional prostaglandin (PG) mediators. Mast cells also have cell-surface receptors for bradykinin. Cellular damage can also induce alterations in normal membrane architecture with the subsequent activation of the complement cascade. Complement component C3a and other inflammatory mediators induce tissue mast cells to degranulate, with the resulting release of histamine and still more inflammatory mediators. Complement component C3b and potentially dead and dying cells that are coated with antibody also stimulate tissue macrophages to release additional inflammatory mediators. Bleeding into the injured tissue increases proteases, which can increase the production of C3b and activate the alternate complement pathway. In addition, fibrinopeptides derived from the clotting cascade have additional stimulatory activity on the tissue macrophages.*

Orchestrating Host Physiology in Response to Antigen

In response to Jimmy's sliver and injured knee, the activities of the immune system are not focused solely on the foreign material or damaged self-structures. The immune system must also coordinate a variety of physiologic responses to prepare the host for the inflammatory response and allow an optimal removal of the offending antigen. A few of the responses induced by Jimmy's injured knee are shown in Fig. 2-3. These activities include the induction of an array of autonomic, behavioral, and metabolic responses. For example, in addition to the entry of fluids into the tissues, the surfaces of endothelial cells in the area of the injury change to allow inflammatory cells to leave the circulation and migrate to the site of injury. Also, a dramatic alteration in the synthetic products of the liver (acute phase response) takes place, production of platelets increases, production of the cells that are being consumed in the inflammatory response increases, and fever is induced. These examples are only a sampling of the physiologic events that are coordinated by the inflammatory response taking place in Jimmy. Therefore, the immune system not only has local effects at the immediate site of the inflammation, but it also has endocrine-like systemic effects at sites distant from the injury.

The preceding section should leave the impression that, at its simplest, the immune system can be thought of as having only two functions: recognizing what does not belong and coordinating the body's other systems in the removal of unwanted materials. This division of labor is a masterpiece of specialization. The antigen-recognition components of this system are incredibly heterogeneous, having the potential to identify and distinguish specifically between molecules and cells that should remain or be removed. Once a structure has been targeted for removal, there are a limited number of biologic activities that the immune system can call upon to aid in its removal. The system is then set up so that an almost infinite number of antigen-binding sites can use a limited number of methods for antigen removal. Generally, the most appropriate method for antigen removal is selected. Two different types of immunity are responsible for this protection: innate immunity and acquired immunity.

FIG. 2-3 ▶

Immune Response Orchestrated at Site of Injury and at Distance from Injury. *The inflammatory mediators produced in response to either a physical trauma or to a foreign antigen have both local and distant activities. Locally, there is a dramatic increase in vascular permeability, and the local endothelial cells express altered cell-adhesion molecules. These structural changes allow phagocytes to leave the circulation and, under the influence of chemotactic factors, migrate to the site of the inflammation. Mediators are also sent to the hypothalamus, which can activate a variety of autonomic and endocrine responses that increase temperature and stimulate the synthesis of stress hormones. The acute phase protein synthesis is stimulated in the liver, and the bone marrow is induced to synthesize more platelets and inflammatory cells. ACTH = adrenocorticotropic hormone.*

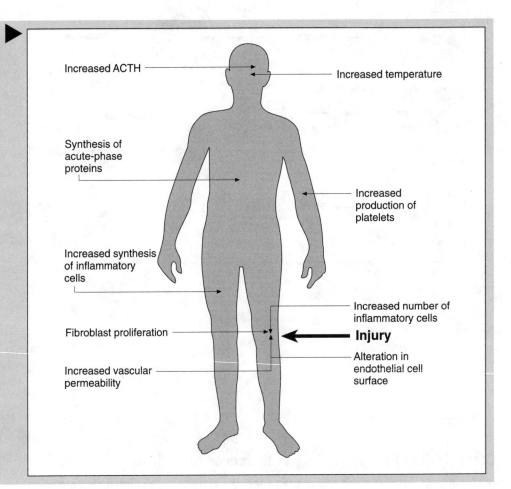

INNATE IMMUNITY

Innate immunity refers to the normal physiologic and anatomic mechanisms of protection. Although innate, or natural, immunity does not have the characteristics of memory and specificity, it is a mistake to view these innate immune functions as independent and separate from the acquired immune response. Natural immune mechanisms limit access to the body, initiate the inflammatory responses, and, in concert with the acquired immune response, eliminate or isolate antigens. Therefore, the response to an antigen ultimately involves not only the acquired response, antibody, and lymphocytes, but also components of natural immunity.

Anatomic Barriers

Innate immunity includes physical barriers to the entrance of pathogens. The skin is an obvious anatomic barrier that in Jimmy was broken, permitting entrance and colonization by bacteria. There are also other anatomic barriers, including the mucous membranes, which can entrap and prevent adherence of bacteria and viruses, and the cilia, which help protect the lungs by removing particulate materials.

Physiologic Barriers

In addition to anatomic barriers, innate immune mechanisms also include physiologic barriers. The acidic environment of the stomach, which inhibits growth of many organisms and can potentially denature nonviable protein antigens, is an example of a physiologic barrier. Elevation of body temperature is also part of natural immunity because the elevated temperature creates an environment that is not optimal for bacterial growth. Other examples of physiologic barriers include the enzymes and proteins in fluids that bathe body surfaces; the lysozyme in tears, which can cleave the cell wall of some organisms; and lactoferrin, which is found in several secretions and which avidly chelates iron and limits access of this nutrient to the local microorganisms.

Phagocytes and Complement

Two components of innate immunity that play central and recurring roles in inflammatory responses are the phagocytic cells and the complement system. To understand the basic concepts of immunology, it is critical to understand the multiple functions of both phagocytic cells and complement.

PHAGOCYTIC CELLS

The term *phagocyte* encompasses a large and diverse population. These cells include monocytes, neutrophils, granulocytes, and a variety of other cells with cytotoxic activity.

Phagocytes perform three different functions. First, they can engulf particles and contain the metabolic machinery to kill viable cells. In this capacity, they are often the first line of defense against infection. However, by themselves, phagocytes cannot distinguish between self- and nonself-antigens. Therefore, the phagocytic cells function together with components of the acquired immune response to identify a foreign structure for removal. Second, phagocytes help initiate antigen-specific reactions. In this capacity, the phagocytes are called antigen-presenting cells (APCs), and they express special cell-surface structures to help them effectively present the antigens and stimulate an antigen-specific acquired immune response. Finally, phagocytes produce an array of cell products that have autocrine, paracrine, and endocrine activities. These phagocytic products coordinate many phases of the immune response, from the initial inflammatory events to the eventual repair of the damaged tissues.

> *Functions of Phagocytic Cells*
> *Remove antigen and kill viable organisms*
> *Present antigen and initiate inflammation*
> *Generate factors to repair the damaged tissues*

COMPLEMENT

In Jimmy's response to both the twisted knee and the sliver, a series of serum proteins called *complement* is identified as playing a central role. The role of the complement system can be thought of in terms of three major activities: (1) initiating the inflammation (anaphylaxis); (2) identifying materials for removal by phagocytic cells (opsonization); and (3) in some cases, lysing a susceptible bacterial cell. How these three functions of complement are related to each other is schematically illustrated in Fig. 2-4.

Figure 2-4 implies that there are three different phases in complement activation: the events in the *initiation* of the complement cascade, the events and reactions that lead to an *amplification* of the complement response, and the events associated with the eventual membrane *lysis*. Although the end products of complement activation—anaphylaxis, opsonization, and lysis—are conceptually simple to understand, the mechanism that the complement system uses to initiate these activities is far more complex and needs to be discussed in more detail.

> *Complement Functions*
> *Anaphylaxis*
> *Opsonization*
> *Lysis*

Classic Complement Pathway. Complement is a complex series of approximately 24 serum proteins. They were initially identified because they work with (complement) the antibody's ability to kill bacteria. Inactive forms (zymogens) of the complement proteins are found in serum. When activated, these proteins eventually lead to the activities outlined in Fig. 2-4.

Central to understanding the biologic role of complement is identifying the two different pathways that are capable of activating the system. One pathway, the *classic*

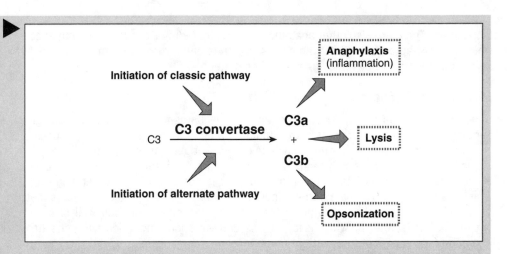

FIG. 2-4

Activities of Complement System. *Complement, a component of innate immunity, is a set of more than 24 serum proteins. These proteins are stored as inactive zymogens in the serum. The activation of complement involves the construction of a protease called C3 convertase. This enzyme splits the serum protein C3 into two very active and important fragments called C3a and C3b. The C3a fragment along with other complement components are anaphylatoxins. Anaphylatoxins cause the activation and degranulation of mast cells, which initiates the inflammatory response. The C3b fragment coats particles and increases their phagocytosis by the local tissue macrophages (opsonization). In addition, C3b helps in the construction of a membrane attack complex that lyses cell membranes. Activated complement also includes factors with other important activities, such as inflammatory cell chemotactic factors. However, the three major functions associated with the complement system are anaphylaxis, opsonization, and lysis.*

complement pathway, depends on specific antibody coating a target (i.e., the acquired immune system is necessary for activation). In this pathway, illustrated in Fig. 2-5, antibody that has bound antigen can react with soluble protein components of the complement system. These initial binding reactions generate proteolytic enzymes that eventually lead to the formation of an enzyme called *C3 convertase*. This reaction is a cascade, analogous to the clotting cascade, in which one initiating event can create several enzymes, each of which is capable of amplifying the signal from the initial binding event. C3 convertase is a protease that converts a serum protein called C3 into two fragments—C3a and C3b. C3 convertase is the central enzyme in the complement system and clearly is playing a major role in Jimmy's response to the bacterial infection because both products of C3 convertase perform important activities in the inflammatory response. C3a is, in part, responsible for the anaphylactic, or inflammatory, activity of the complement system. C3b can bind covalently to surfaces and is responsible for marking materials for removal by phagocytes (opsonization). The C3 convertase itself can be modified by reaction with additional C3b to begin a series of interactions that eventually lead to the formation of a membrane attack complex, which results in cell lysis.

This classic method of activating the complement system is absolutely dependent

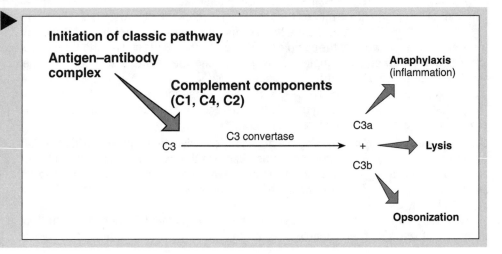

FIG. 2-5

Activation of Classic Complement Pathway. *The complement system and its resulting activities can be activated by two independent pathways. Both pathways result in the formation of the enzyme C3 convertase. The classic complement pathway has an absolute requirement for antigen–antibody complexes and, as such, requires a successful acquired immune response. In addition, complement factors C1, C4, and C2 are components of this pathway.*

on antibody and, as such, requires antibody and the acquired immune response prior to activation of the complement. Antibody to foreign antigens, such as the materials on Jimmy's sliver, will activate this system. In addition, antibody to dead, dying, or modified self-cells can also activate the classic complement pathway with the resulting inflammation, opsonization, and potential cell lysis.

Alternate Complement Pathway. Jimmy's other injury, his twisted knee, allowed no introduction of foreign substances, and therefore, there were potentially no antigen–antibody complexes available to initiate the complement system via the classic pathway. In this case, an alternate method exists to create the enzyme C3 convertase. This second activation pathway, the *alternate complement pathway*, is independent of the acquired immune response and provides a unique method for distinguishing between self- and either foreign or altered self-molecules.

The activation of the alternate complement pathway is a continuous process (Fig. 2-6). Under the influence of serum and tissue proteases, serum complement component C3 is slowly cleaved to form low levels of the products C3a and C3b. This is the same reaction catalyzed by C3 convertase. The C3b formed by the reaction with protease can bind to an additional serum factor—factor B—that through the action of another complement protease—factor D—produces an alternate form of the enzyme C3 convertase. As discussed earlier, the enzyme C3 convertase dramatically increases the production of both C3a and C3b and causes an explosive increase in the rate of complement activation with high levels of all complement products. Without mechanisms to interfere with this activation, the complement system would be continuously activating inflammation and consuming all of the serum complement components. To prevent this nonspecific activation, there are serum factors that compete with the alternate activation pathway. Two of

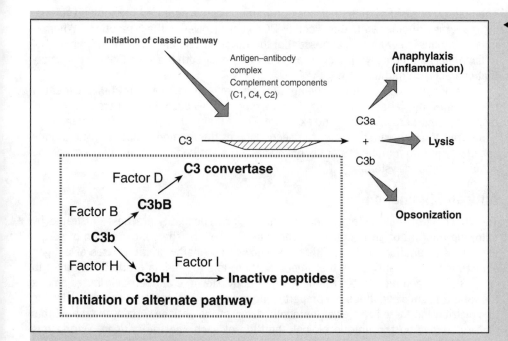

◄ **FIG. 2-6**
Activation of Alternate Complement Pathway. *The complement system and its resulting activities can be activated by two independent pathways. Both pathways result in the formation of the enzyme C3 convertase. The alternate complement pathway does not require antigen–antibody complexes and, therefore, can be initiated rapidly in response to tissue damage or to an infecting microorganism. The alternate pathway requires a surface that stabilizes C3 convertase. Under the influence of tissue proteases and clotting enzymes, serum C3 is constantly being broken down into components C3a and C3b. There is then a competition for the C3b that is being generated. The C3b can either react with factor B and be processed by factor D to form C3 convertase, if there is a stabilizing surface, or the C3b can react with factor H and be processed by factor I to form inactive peptides. In the presence of a stabilizing surface or increased production of C3b, a C3 convertase is generated. In the absence of a stabilizing surface and normal C3b production, factors H and I are more effective competitors, and there is inactivation of the C3b that was formed. It is important to note that mammalian cells contain factors that make them unsuitable surfaces for activation of the alternate pathway. However, some bacteria are excellent inducers of the alternate pathway because they lack the components that destabilize the alternate pathway C3 convertase.*

these factors, factor H and factor I, are also illustrated in Fig. 2-6. The serum factor H binds to the C3b and, under the influence of factor I, the C3bH complex is irreversibly destroyed. In this situation, factors B and H compete for the available C3b. When low levels of C3b are generated, factor H is an excellent competitor for the available C3b, and there is no net complement activation. In addition to factor H competition for C3b, mammalian cells have developed mechanisms that destabilize the activated C3bBb complement components on the cell surface.

The alternate complement pathway is, then, a system that is constantly starting and being turned off. An equilibrium is established that depends on a slow consistent generation of C3b, the interaction of C3b and factor B on an unstable surface, and competition for the available C3b by factors H and I. All of these factors lead to a net inactivation of complement. However, if the normal physiology changes, such that increased C3b is generated (e.g., bleeding, tissue damage) or a surface is introduced that stabilizes the C3 convertase (e.g., a bacterial cell or damaged self-tissues), then the serum inhibitors factors H and I are poor competitors, and the alternate complement pathway is activated.

Once activated by either the classic or alternate pathways, complement product C3b can opsonize cells and particles for removal by the phagocytic cells, and component C3a and other complement fragments with anaphylactic activity trigger the inflammatory response. All of these innate immune events happened in response to both of Jimmy's injuries.

ACQUIRED IMMUNITY

The major focus of any course or book on immunology is acquired immunity. Lymphocytes are the principal white blood cell (WBC) types involved in these reactions. Whereas innate immune mechanisms are essential for initiation of inflammation and removal of inflammatory antigens, lymphocytes are responsible for both the specificity and memory that characterize immunology.

The acquired component of the immune system includes both the ability to identify the foreign material and the ability to remember a previously encountered agent and respond more vigorously on second exposure. This enhanced response to foreign material is referred to as the anamnestic, the secondary, or the memory response. The unique specificity of the immune system is provided by the antibodies and lymphocytes of the acquired immune system.

Antigen Elimination

The concepts of immunologic memory and antigen specificity are best illustrated by following the fate of an injected antigen. Fig. 2-7 follows the concentration of serum antigen as a function of time. This curve shows four characteristic phases of antigen elimination. When antigen is first injected, there is an immediate dilutional effect in which the antigen distributes throughout the body. How the antigen distributes among the various tissues and fluids is a property unique to each antigen. Immediately following this distribution there is a slower metabolic decay of the antigen. Again, the rate of this decay depends on the unique biologic half-life of each specific antigen. During this period, the antigen is available to the immune system and is activating components of the acquired immune system. Once the immune system has been activated, cells and antibody capable of binding the antigen are generated. These factors then rapidly react with the free antigen and remove it from the circulation. These events are illustrated in the third, or antigen elimination, phase (Fig. 2-7). It is important to note that free antibody cannot be easily detected during this period because the free antibody removes any available antigen. Only when the free antigen is removed is it possible to detect specific antibody easily. In this fourth phase of the antigen elimination curve, after free antigen is removed, an excess of free antibody can be detected.

Fig. 2-7 also shows that the curve changes if the acquired immune system has memory of a previous encounter with the identical antigen. In this case, the metabolic

Phases of Antigen Elimination
Dilution and tissue distribution
Metabolic decay
Immune elimination
Antibody excess

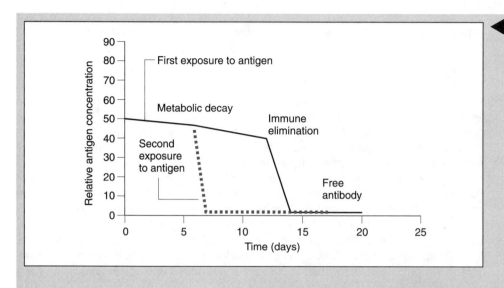

FIG. 2-7
Antigen Elimination Curve. *When antigen is injected and the blood concentration of antigen is followed as a function of time, there are four characteristic phases in the resulting curve. Initially, there is a rapid dilution and distribution of the antigen throughout the body. Following this initial dilution, the antigen concentration slowly decays with a half-life that is characteristic for each unique antigen. During this period, the immune system is being stimulated. For the first exposure to antigen, this period can last 12–18 days. Once the immune system has been stimulated, there is a rapid immunologic elimination of antigen. It is during this immune elimination phase that there are circulating antigen-antibody immune complexes. Following the elimination of antigen, free antibody can be detected in the circulation. If the individual was previously exposed to the identical antigen, the metabolic decay period is significantly reduced, and antigen is eliminated faster.*

decay phase of the antigen elimination curve is significantly shortened. When there is a significant amount of previously formed antibody, there may be no detectable period between antigen infection and immune elimination. To observe this memory response, the previous exposure requires the identical antigen. This is an illustration of the specificity of the immune response. A nonrelated antigen cannot induce memory. Similar primary and secondary immune responses are seen when either antibody (humoral) or lymphocyte (cell-mediated) responses are evaluated.

The primary and secondary responses differ not only in terms of kinetics (see Fig. 2-7) but also in magnitude. When evaluating the antibody component of the immune system, the type of antibody produced differs between the primary and secondary immune responses. Fig. 2-8 illustrates this point. In this figure, the difference in magnitude between the primary and secondary response is clearly evident. Also illustrated are differences in the type of antibody molecules that are produced. Immunoglobulin M (IgM) antibody is observed in primary responses, whereas IgG, IgE, and IgA antibodies are observed in secondary responses. The term *isotype* refers to these differ-

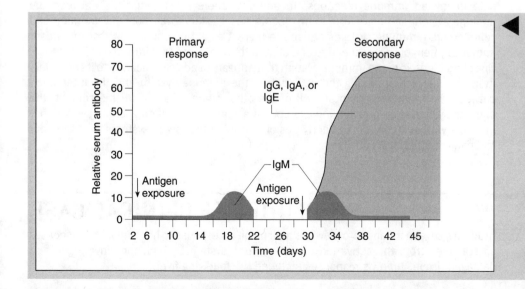

FIG. 2-8
Comparison of Primary and Secondary Antibody Responses. *The primary and secondary antibody responses differ from each other both qualitatively and quantitatively. The primary response generally requires 12–18 days and predominantly consists of the IgM antibody. During this primary response, the immune system is developing memory and the ability to respond with other antibody isotypes should there be a second exposure to the antigen. Upon secondary exposure to the antigen, there is again an IgM response; however, this time the IgM response happens much more rapidly, and it is overwhelmed by the magnitude of either an IgG, IgE, or IgA response.*

ent antibody classes. Therefore, the primary and the secondary antibody responses differ from each other both quantitatively and qualitatively.

Cellular and Humoral Immunity

As identified above, acquired immunity is most often separated into two different systems: humoral immunity and cellular immunity. Both cellular and humoral immunity depend on the activation of a type of WBC called a *lymphocyte*. This division between the humoral and cell-mediated immune systems is illustrated in Fig. 2-9. Antibody synthesized by plasma cells that have differentiated from B lymphocytes is central to humoral immune responses. Cellular immunity, on the other hand, includes those immune reactions that are mediated by T lymphocytes, of which there are multiple types. At this stage only two different populations of T cells are discussed—helper T lymphocytes (Th lymphocytes) and cytotoxic T lymphocytes (Tc lymphocytes). Much of the study of immunology involves expanding Fig. 2-9 and elucidating in far more detail how humoral (B-cell) and cell-mediated (Th cells and Tc cells) immunity produce immunologic memory and antigenic specificity, the hallmarks of the acquired immune system.

FIG. 2-9

Components of Acquired Immunity. *The acquired immune response is comprised of humoral (antibody) immunity and cell-mediated immunity. In humoral immune mechanisms, B lymphocytes are stimulated to differentiate into plasma cells, which secrete antibodies of either IgM (primary immune response) or IgG, IgE, or IgA (secondary immune response) isotypes. Antibody eliminates antigen by aggregation (agglutination or precipitation), opsonization, lytic mechanisms, detoxification, or limiting access of the antigen. Cell-mediated immunity is the domain of T lymphocytes, and antigen is eliminated by delayed-type hypersensitivity reactions or by cytotoxic T lymphocytes (Tc). Th = helper T lymphocytes.*

Acquired Immune Response

Humoral immunity	**Cell-mediated immunity**
(IgM, IgG, IgE, IgA; B lymphocytes)	(Th,Tc lymphocytes)
Aggregation (complement, phagocytes)	Delayed hypersensitivity (Th lymphocytes)
Opsonization (complement, phagocytes)	Cytotoxic T cells (Tc lymphocytes)
Lysis (complement)	
Detoxification	
Limit access	

As any course in immunology unfolds, it should become clear that dividing the immune system into the isolated components of T cells and antibody is an artificial division. Cells, antibody, and soluble factors produced by cells (i.e., cytokines) participate in myriad immune reactions. In addition, there are interactions between the immune system and cells from nonlymphoid tissues. Moreover, both the humoral and cell-mediated immune systems depend to a great extent on components of the innate immune system both to respond to and eliminate the antigen that initiated the response. One characteristic of the immune system that appears to add significantly to its complexity is the interaction among the cells within the immune system and the interaction between the immune system and all of the other organ systems. In this context, the immune system is an outstanding example of a super-, or regulatory, organ system that interacts with and controls the activities of multiple other organ systems that carry out mechanical functions.

RESOLUTION OF CLINICAL CASE

In Jimmy, several inflammatory events took place in response to his injury. The responses all stemmed from the activation of the immune system by both foreign antigen and damaged tissue. Jimmy's responses included the following five:

- **Recognition.** Jimmy's two injuries were clearly different in that one involved the introduction of foreign material, whereas the other involved no foreign antigen with access to the second site. However, the resulting inflammatory responses were similar for both injuries. In the case of the sliver of wood, foreign materials were introduced into the wound. If this had been the second exposure to these foreign materials, then preformed antibody could have coated the foreign particle and activated the classic complement pathway. The antibody or complement-coated particles would then have been targets for phagocytic cells.

  In the case of the damaged knee, no foreign materials were introduced. However, cells had been damaged and cell surfaces altered, which primed the immune system to mark dead or dying cells for removal. Consequently, the damaged cells may also have been marked with antibody. In the absence of a specific antibody, however, both injuries introduced new surfaces into the body that promoted the alternate complement pathway. Moreover, either introducing the sliver or damaging the knee likely resulted in bleeding, which activates the clotting mechanism. The increased number of proteases resulting from the activation of the clotting cascade can also act on local complement component C3, producing increased quantities of C3a and C3b, again promoting the activation of the alternate complement pathway.

- **Recruiting Inflammatory Cells.** Inflammatory cells need to be recruited to the area of the tissue injury. The C3a from the complement system, either the classic pathway or the alternate pathway, stimulates inflammation. In addition, factors from the damaged cells and the activated clotting system can activate the local tissue macrophages. Antibody and C3b-opsonized materials also act as potent activators of the tissue macrophages. The activated macrophages then secrete additional inflammatory cytokines.

- **Removal of Foreign or Damaged Material.** The inflammatory cells infiltrating the area are able to phagocytize antibody and C3b-coated materials. If these materials include living cells, such as bacteria, the inflammatory cells have the capability of using extremely toxic chemical agents to kill the unwanted cell. Because of the potency of these chemicals, it is not unexpected that there is collateral damage to healthy host structures. This damage to healthy tissue is called a *hypersensitivity reaction*, and it is a consequence of the immune response. In some cases, the pathology of a disease is more closely related to damage caused by the immune response than to the tissue damage caused by the organism.

- **Establishing Immunologic Memory.** The result of a local inflammatory reaction produces soluble or cellular debris from the target antigen. The antigen structures can then be moved through the lymphatic system, where they can initiate lymphocyte reactions that culminate in a memory of the immune response.

- **Repair of Damaged Tissue.** In an additional activity, the activated macrophages produce factors that promote growth and repair of the damaged tissue, both that caused by the initial tissue injury as well as that caused by the immune response to the injury.

REVIEW QUESTIONS

Directions: For each of the following questions, choose the **one best** answer.

1. Which one of the following phrases describes an example of a mechanism of innate immunity?

   (A) Antibody opsonization of bacteria

   (B) Inhibition of bacterial colonization activities of the ciliated mucosa of the bronchial tree

   (C) T lymphocyte response to a vaccine

   (D) Elimination of antigen by the formation of an antigen–antibody complex

   (E) Killing of a target cell by an activated T lymphocyte

2. Which one of the following statements correctly describes differences between the primary and secondary immune responses?

   (A) A secondary immune response is observed only in humoral (antibody) immunity.

   (B) The primary immune response is higher in magnitude but takes longer to develop than the secondary response.

   (C) The primary immune response is lower in magnitude and takes longer to develop than the secondary immune response.

   (D) The secondary immune response is lower in magnitude and takes longer to develop than the primary immune response.

3. Which one of the following statements describes the differences between the classic and alternate complement pathways?

   (A) Although the classic and alternate pathways are initiated differently, similar mechanisms are available for amplification and lysis by components of the system.

   (B) Only the classic complement pathway involves the generation of the enzyme C3 convertase.

   (C) Antibody is required for the activity of both the classic and alternate complement pathways.

   (D) The alternate complement pathway allows bacterial lysis, whereas the classic pathway promotes anaphylaxis and opsonization.

4. Which one of the following tissues or locations is exempt from the immune system's ability to detect antigen?

   (A) Interstitial fluid

   (B) Heart

   (C) Liver

   (D) Inside of a red blood cell that is not making proteins

5. A patient suffered a total blockage in a major artery of the heart. As a result, a section of the heart died and became necrotic from the lack of oxygen. Because no foreign organisms were introduced, which one of the following statements best describes the immune response to this sterile, necrotic tissue?

   (A) There will be no inflammatory response.

   (B) Because the tissue is sterile, only the B-cell component of the immune system will be able to respond.

   (C) Because the tissue is sterile, only the T-cell component of the immune system will be able to respond.

   (D) Although there are inflammatory responses, they are nonspecific and do not involve cells of the immune system.

   (E) Components of the immune system detect dead and damaged autologous tissues and initiate inflammatory responses similar to inflammation caused by foreign antigens.

6. Which one of the following statements best describes the interactions between the immune system and other organ systems?

   (A) The immune system is totally isolated from all other organ systems.

   (B) Immune responses can alter the activities and functions of the organ system involved in an inflammatory process; however, the immune system will not affect the activities of organ systems that are not infected.

   (C) Although the immune system can alter the responses of other organ systems, the effects are local and affect only organs surrounding the inflammatory site.

   (D) The immune system can alter the responses of multiple organ systems both local and distant to the inflammatory site.

   (E) Although cells and other components of the immune system can be found in all organs and tissues, immune responses have no effect on nonlymphoid tissues.

7. An example of a complement-mediated activity is

   (A) antibody production

   (B) initiation of inflammation

   (C) activation of B lymphocytes

   (D) killing of a target cell by T lymphocytes

   (E) acute phase response of the liver

8. Lymphocytes and phagocytes must interact and function to produce the most effective response to a foreign agent. Which one of the following functions is uniquely associated with the lymphocytes?

   (A) Distinguishing between self and foreign materials

   (B) Killing infecting organisms

   (C) Presenting antigens to the immune system

   (D) Synthesizing factors to repair damaged tissues

   (E) Synthesizing factors to coordinate inflammatory activities

9. The alternate and classic complement pathways differ in which one of the following ways?

   (A) The mechanism of cell lysis

   (B) The mediators that trigger inflammation

   (C) The mechanisms of initiating complement activation

   (D) The necessity of the enzyme C3 convertase

ANSWERS AND EXPLANATIONS

1. **The answer is B.** Normal physiologic processes that limit bacterial growth or prevent bacterial or antigen access are parts of the natural immune system. The activities of the ciliated mucosa of the bronchial tree, in inhibiting bacterial colonization, prevent bacterial access to the lung and are an example of this mechanism. The antibody responses of B lymphocytes and the activities of T lymphocytes are part of the acquired immune response.

2. **The answer is C.** Upon first exposure, there are limited numbers of cells capable of responding to any antigen. During this first exposure, it is necessary for antigen-specific T and B lymphocytes to interact. The responding cells then must proliferate and prepare the proper type of response for the nature of the antigen and the route of antigen exposure. Upon secondary exposure to antigen, there are significantly more cells capable of responding, and the requirement for cells to interact with each other is significantly minimized.

3. **The answer is A.** Both the classic and alternate complement pathways have an absolute requirement for the enzyme C3 convertase. This enzyme is necessary to make C3a, an anaphylatoxin; C3b, an opsonin; and the membrane attack complex, which results in lysis of susceptible cells. Different proteins make up the alternate pathway C3 convertase and the classic pathway C3 convertase. The different proteins reflect differences in the initiation of the classic and alternate pathways. The classic pathway is initiated by antibody–antigen complexes, whereas the alternate pathway is initiated by both increased nonspecific production of C3b and a foreign surface that can stabilize the alternate pathway C3 convertase.

4. **The answer is D.** The immune system functions to survey the metabolic products of all nucleated cells and tissues and must have access to each of the organ systems. There are only a few tissues that are considered immunologically privileged sites, meaning that the immune system has limited or no access to the tissue. These privileged sites include the inside of the red blood cell (no proteins are being synthesized) and the anterior chamber of the eye.

5. **The answer is E.** Even if dead or dying tissues are sterile, it is possible for them to induce an inflammatory response. One role of the immune system is to mark dead and dying tissues for removal, and the immune system contains antibodies to identify tissues expressing altered or abnormal surface molecules. In addition, the alternate pathway of complement can be activated by cell surfaces that have lost the normal mechanisms to inactivate the C3 convertase.

6. **The answer is D.** The immune system is capable of altering the functional activity of cells in the location of an inflammatory response. In addition, the immune system has endocrine-like activities in which an inflammatory response is able to alter the activities of tissues and organs that are at sites distant from the inflammation. The fever response and the acute phase protein response are two examples in which the immune response dramatically alters the activity of distant organ systems.

7. **The answer is B.** The complement system can be thought of as a method to call in rapidly the immune system (i.e., it initiates inflammation). As a result of this inflammation, B lymphocytes can be activated, antibody can be produced, T lymphocytes can kill target cells, and the responses of multiple distant tissues can be altered.

8. **The answer is A.** In all but a few cases, the macrophage and other phagocytic cells cannot distinguish between self- and nonself-structures. Macrophages slowly and continually sample the environment. If, however, the cell encounters a structure that

is coated with antibody, the macrophage has a cell membrane receptor for a portion of the antibody and rapidly engulfs opsonized materials. Some bacteria contain cell wall components (e.g., lipopolysaccharides) that activate the macrophage to increase the rate of phagocytosis of all materials in the environment. However, even in this case, the phagocytic cell cannot distinguish self- from nonself-structures.

9. **The answer is C.** Antigen–antibody complexes activate the classic pathway of complement. Stabilizing surfaces or structures activate the alternate pathway, which can be activated rapidly in response to some bacteria because there is no dependence on an initial antibody response.

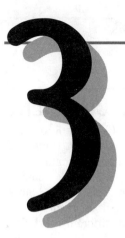

CELLS AND TISSUES OF THE IMMUNE SYSTEM

INTRODUCTION OF CLINICAL CASE

Sarah, a 12-year-old girl, was brought to her primary care provider by her mother. For the past 2 days, Sarah has had a fever and a sore throat. Sarah's general appearance was that of a sick, uncomfortable child. Upon examination, Sarah's physician found several hard, swollen lymph nodes in her neck. In addition, an examination of Sarah's throat revealed an erythematous mucosa with numerous whitish patches, red swollen tonsils, and a significant amount of exudate. A rapid microbiologic analysis from Sarah's throat revealed a significant number of streptococcal organisms. A white blood cell (WBC) count with differential was also ordered, and the results are presented in Table 3-1.

TABLE 3-1 ▶

Sarah's White Blood Cell (WBC) Count with Differential

	Sarah	*Normal Values*
WBC count	$18 \times 10^3/\mu L$	$7–14 \times 10^3/\mu L$
Segmented neutrophils	74%	60%–70%
Banded neutrophils	1%	0%–5%
Lymphocytes	20%	20%–40%
Monocytes	4%	2%–6%
Basophils	0%	0%–1%
Eosinophils	1%	1%–4%

LEUKOCYTE ONTOGENY

Basic Concept of Immunology
All cells needed for a successful immune response are derived from a single bone marrow pluripotent stem cell.

The term **leukocyte** refers to all WBCs.

The white cells listed in the complete blood count (CBC) in Table 3-1 are derived in the bone marrow from a single pluripotent precursor cell called a *stem cell*. Under the influence of the appropriate growth and differentiation factors, the self-replicating stem cells can be influenced to proliferate and differentiate into any of the cells listed in Sarah's WBC count. In addition to the WBCs (leukocytes) listed in Table 3-1, red blood cells (RBCs) and platelets also are derived from the same bone marrow precursor cell. Fig. 3-1 illustrates the developmental relationship between these different cell types. Generally, the intermediate cells along any pathway are seldom seen in the blood, and when they are observed in the peripheral circulation, it is generally an indication of pathology. One of the fundamental concepts of immunology is that the cells needed for a successful immune response are derived from this single pluripotent stem cell produced in bone marrow.

FIGURE 3-1 ▶

Ontogeny of the Immune System. *All of the cells that make up the immune system are derived from a single, pluripotent, bone-marrow–derived stem cell. The stem cell makes progenitor cells of the granulocytes, monocytes, and lymphocytes. Under the influence of the appropriate growth and differentiation factors, these progenitor cells can differentiate into each of the cells identified in this figure. The stem cell is also the precursor to red blood cells and platelets.*

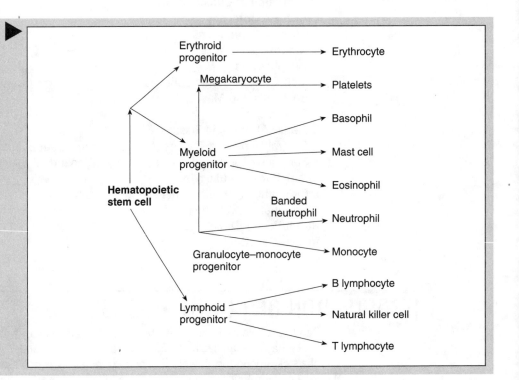

LEUKOCYTE POPULATIONS

The leukocyte population reported in Sarah's WBC count lists several morphologically different cells (see Table 3-1). Although all of the cells have a common origin in the bone marrow, they have different structures and different functional roles in the inflammatory response. In Sarah's case, most of the cell populations reported in the WBC count are within the normal range; however, the neutrophil population is significantly elevated. When the immune system responds to an infection, the type of cell responding is generally able to provide a clue to the nature of the infectious agent. In Sarah's case, the immune response to the infecting organism is sending the necessary signals to increase the number of neutrophils to fight the infection. To understand how the immune system responds to and removes antigen, it is necessary to understand the nature, structure, and function of each type of leukocyte.

Neutrophils

The neutrophil is a phagocytic leukocyte and is the most abundant type. The terms *polymorphonuclear neutrophil (PMN)* and *segmented neutrophil* are used interchangeably to refer to this cell type. The latter term is derived from the multilobed nature of the cell's nucleus (Fig. 3-2). Generally, neutrophil nuclei exhibit 3–5 segmented lobes. A second characteristic of functional importance to the cell is the large number of cytoplasmic granules. These granules contain acid hydrolases, such as proteases, nucleases, glycosidases, and the enzyme myeloperoxidase. Neutrophils are also rich in the enzymes and metabolic pathways necessary for the production and use of reactive oxygen species (e.g., hydrogen peroxide, superoxide, hydroxyl radical). Given this battery of toxic granule contents, it is easy to identify a major function for the neutrophils. Neutrophils are efficient killing cells that can use their toxic oxygen molecules to lyse microorganisms and digest biologic molecules. This cell type and its regulation are amazing. Billions of neutrophils are synthesized and released from the bone marrow each day, making it one of the most dynamic cell types in the body. Neutrophils are directed toward the site of inflammatory reactions by critical signaling molecules called *cytokines*. When stimulated by the appropriate cytokine, neutrophils leave the circulation and enter the inflamed tissue, carry out their function, and then die. Once in the tissues, the neutrophils do not leave to re-enter the circulation. If a circulating neutrophil is not used within 1 week, the cell dies and must be replaced.

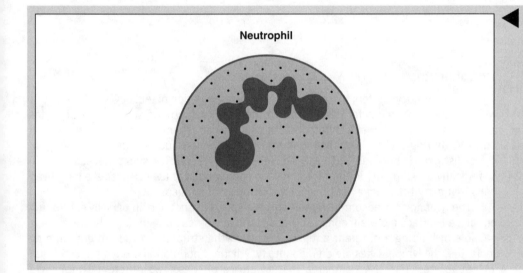

Neutrophil

FIGURE 3-2

Segmented Neutrophils. Neutrophils (segmented neutrophils; polymorphonuclear neutrophils) are phagocytic cells with a multilobed nucleus and prominent cytoplasmic granules. The cell expresses Fc receptors for antibody and receptors for the C3b component of complement, which allows the neutrophil to identify the target of the acquired immune response. The cytoplasmic granules of the neutrophil contain hydrolytic enzymes and myeloperoxidase. Moreover, the cells generate active oxygen species and use their toxic granule contents to kill bacteria and clear necrotic tissues.

Although the neutrophil is capable of killing microorganisms, the cell itself does not contain the information necessary to differentiate between host cells and cells or organisms that do not belong. Consequently, the killing function of the cell must be carefully regulated to prevent damaging important normal self-structures. It is the job of the acquired immune system to mark foreign materials for removal by the neutrophil. To accomplish this task, the neutrophil expresses cell-surface receptors that specifically bind to antibody and the C3b component of complement. In this manner, the neutrophil can be directed to kill specific antibody or complement-coated target. Because of the lytic nature of its granule contents, the neutrophil is uniquely suited to kill bacteria and is most often associated with the humoral immune response to bacteria or necrotic tissues. Elevations in blood neutrophils are generally seen early in an immune response and in acute immunologic reactions.

Banded Neutrophil. Like segmented neutrophil, the term *banded neutrophil* is derived from the cell's characteristic nuclear staining. In this case, however, instead of a multilobed, segmented nucleus, the nuclear material is in a simple U-shaped pattern (Fig. 3-3). The banded neutrophil is an immature cell on the way to becoming a mature, segmented neutrophil. When there is demand for neutrophils because of an infection or chronic cell damage, the bone marrow is stimulated to release its supply of mature (segmented) and some immature (banded) cells. Generally, in the presence of a long-term bacterial infection or chronic tissue necrosis, the level of "bands" reported in the CBC increases.

FIGURE 3-3 ▶

Banded Neutrophil. Banded neutrophils (bands) are immature segmented neutrophils. Unlike the mature cells, their nucleus takes on a characteristic banded or U-shaped staining pattern. An increase in the number of banded neutrophils usually indicates a prolonged demand for the segmented neutrophil and a call to the bone marrow to release the cells as soon as they are formed.

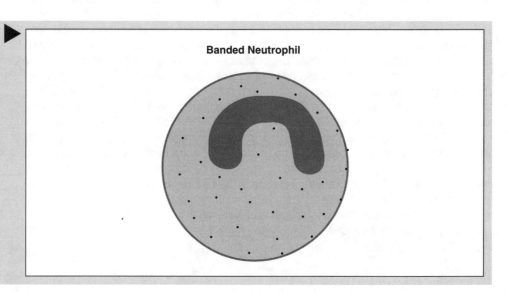

Banded Neutrophil

Lymphocytes

The term lymphocyte refers to a large and complex population of leukocytes, the study of which is the major focus for learning about the acquired immune system. Lymphocytes are the smallest of the leukocyte populations. The cell is almost entirely nucleus with only a slight ring of cytoplasm that contains no prominent vacuoles or granules. Lymphocytes distinguish between self- and nonself-structures and, as such, are essential in specifically directing the immune response to each unique antigen. These are long-lived cells that carry the memory of previously encountered antigens.

Antigen specificity of the immune response and immunologic memory are due entirely to the lymphocytes.

The lymphocytes accomplish their antigen-specific functions, in part, by expressing on the cell surface a protein complex that specifically binds antigen. Each lymphocyte is capable of binding a different antigen. Based on the structure of the antigen-binding molecule, the lymphocytes are divided into two distinct populations: B lymphocytes and T lymphocytes. Fig. 3-4 compares the structures of these two different lymphocyte receptors for antigen.

The B-lymphocyte antigen receptor is a membrane-bound version of the immunoglobulin M (IgM) antibody molecule. The carboxy-terminal domain of the antibody, however, is embedded in the lymphocyte membrane, whereas the section of the molecule that reacts with antigen is exposed on the surface of the cell. Lymphocytes expressing membrane-bound IgM antibody are defined as B lymphocytes. Accompanied by its antigen receptor, a B cell is schematically illustrated in Fig. 3-5. B lymphocytes are the precursors to the antibody-forming plasma cells and, therefore, play a central role in humoral or antibody immunity.

In addition to the structural differences between the antigen-binding receptors, T lymphocytes differ from B lymphocytes in a number of important areas. Whereas B lymphocytes are central in humoral (antibody) immunity, the T lymphocytes play multiple roles, both in cell-mediated immunity as well as helping B lymphocytes differentiate into plasma cells. One clear structural difference between B lymphocytes and T lymphocytes is in the nature of the T lymphocyte's receptor for antigen. Although the T-cell antigen receptor (TCR) is a member of the antibody superfamily of molecules, the receptor is somewhat smaller than the IgM molecule found on B lymphocytes. The TCR is further complicated by an associated series of proteins that are necessary to transmit the

Immunoglobulin Superfamily
Certain structural elements of proteins have proved successful and consequently are used repeatedly in multiple protein structures. The immunoglobulin fold or domain is one such structural protein motif. Proteins that incorporate this folding motif are identified as being in the immunoglobulin superfamily. The term, however, implies no functional similarity.

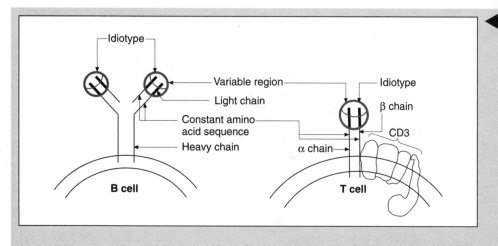

FIGURE 3-4
B- and T- Lymphocyte Antigen Receptors.
The antigen specificity of the immune system is due to both the B-cell receptor for antigen and the T-cell receptor (TCR) for antigen. These antigen receptors can be viewed as constructed of two parts: a structural part that exhibits a constant amino acid sequence from one cell to the other and a variable sequence that is unique for each different cell. It is the variable sequence that uniquely binds antigen. The light and heavy chains of the antibody and the α and β chains of the TCR contain the antigen-binding site. This antigen-binding part of the receptor is called the idiotype. Reagents that bind to the constant part of the receptor can be used to identify all B cells or all T cells. Reagents that bind to the idiotype of the receptor can be used to identify unique antigen-binding specificity. The TCR also consists of a set of proteins called the CD3 molecules, which are necessary for signal transduction. The CD3 molecules are also a constant part of the TCR, and reagents that bind to the CD3 molecules can be used to identify all T cells.

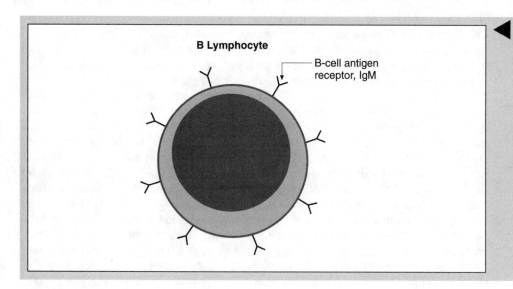

FIGURE 3-5
B Lymphocyte. The antigen receptor on the B lymphocyte is a membrane IgM molecule. B lymphocytes are the precursors of both plasma cells and memory cells. Once stimulated, B lymphocytes, with help from T lymphocytes, will proliferate and differentiate into plasma cells or memory cells. Plasma cells produce and secrete antibody of the identical idiotype that was on the parent B lymphocyte. B cells are therefore critical in antibody or humoral immunity.

signal generated when an antigen has bound to the TCR. This set of associated signal transduction molecules is called the *CD3 complex.*

Whereas the variable portion of the TCR is different for each unique antigen, the CD3 complex has a constant structure from one T cell to the next. The presence of the CD3 molecule then uniquely defines the T lymphocyte and distinguishes it from the B lymphocyte. A schematic illustration of the T lymphocyte is shown in Fig. 3-6. It is important to point out that B and T lymphocytes cannot be distinguished microscopically. Distinguishing between B and T lymphocytes requires special staining techniques that detect either B-lymphocyte IgM (cell-surface IgM) or a TCR.

Lymphocytes also carry the memory of a previous antigen encounter and are, then, very different from the neutrophils discussed previously. Not only are lymphocytes long-lived cells, they also have the capability of entering and leaving body tissues. Moreover,

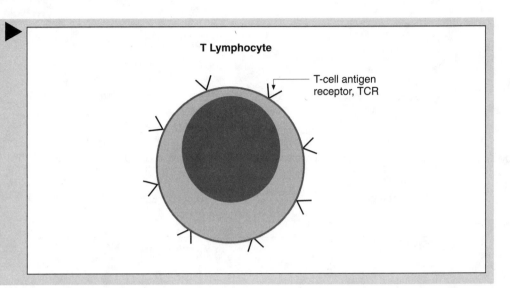

FIGURE 3-6 ▶

T Lymphocyte. *T lymphocytes are small, round leukocytes with a large nucleus-to-cytoplasm ratio that express an antigen receptor different from the B-cell surface immunoglobulin. The receptor for antigen is called the T-cell receptor (TCR). Microscopically, T cells and B cells look identical. These two cell types are distinguished by the nature of the antigen receptor. T cells have multiple functions, and there are multiple populations of T cells that are associated with each of the functions. T cells help B cells make antibody. In addition, T cells are important regulatory and effector cells of the immune response. They participate in cytotoxic reactions and mediate a type of reaction called delayed-type hypersensitivity.*

unlike neutrophils and the other cell types, lymphocytes, when supplied with the appropriate growth and differentiation factors, can proliferate and differentiate into other cell types, such as plasma cells and memory cells.

At this point, only two different populations of lymphocytes have been considered—B cells and T cells. The functions of the T-lymphocyte populations comprise a major component of the study of the immune system. As the functional differences between different T lymphocytes become more apparent, different subpopulations of the cells also become evident.

Cell Differentiation Nomenclature. Morphologically, all lymphocytes look similar using most classic staining procedures. Most lymphocytes are small, round cells with a high nucleus-to-cytoplasmic ratio. Some lymphocytes are "activated," as evidenced by a larger cell size and more cytoplasm. However, differences between B and T cells or between different subsets of T cells cannot be distinguished based on traditional staining techniques. Making the distinction between B and T cells or different subpopulations of T cells depends on the presence or absence of cell-surface molecular structures that are unique to each cell type. These cell-surface structures that differ among cell populations are called *differentiation antigens*. For example, lymphocyte IgM is a unique differentiation antigen for the B-cell population, and the TCR is a unique differentiation antigen for the T-cell population. These differentiation antigens are detected by making antibody reagents (monoclonal antibodies) that uniquely bind to a single differentiation antigen. When reagents from several different research laboratories identify or cluster around the same cell-surface structure, this cluster of differentiation antigens is identified with a unique cell differentiation (CD) number. Therefore, each CD number defines a different functional unit on a cell surface. For example, CD3 defines the set of proteins that helps signal an antigen-binding event on T lymphocytes. Therefore, all T lymphocytes express the CD3 differentiation antigens. Helper T (Th) lymphocytes express the CD4 differentiation antigen, whereas cytotoxic T lymphocytes (CTLs) express the CD8 differentiation antigen.

Monocytes and Macrophages

Several different names are used to discuss the monocyte and macrophage populations. Cells in the monocyte and macrophage population found in the circulation are appropriately called *monocytes*. When the monocytes have migrated into a tissue, the term *histiocyte* or *macrophage* is appropriate. Histiocytes in each of the different organs or tissues are also referred to by a name unique to that tissue. For example, macrophages found in the skin are called Langerhans' cells. However, if the cell were found in the liver, it would be called a Kupffer's cell. The term dendritic cell is often, but not always, used to refer to macrophages found in lymphoid tissues. Table 3-2 provides a list of examples of macrophages and antigen-presenting cells.

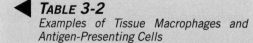
TABLE 3-2
Examples of Tissue Macrophages and Antigen-Presenting Cells

Tissue	Macrophage
Blood	Monocyte
Tissue	Histiocyte or macrophage
Skin	Langerhans' cell
Liver	Kupffer's cell
Lymphoid tissue	Dendritic cell
Connective tissue	Histiocyte
Kidney	Mesangial cell
Brain	Microglial cell
Lung	Alveolar macrophage

A schematic illustration of the circulating monocyte is depicted in Fig. 3-7. This phagocytic cell often has a bilobed or U-shaped nucleus. It has significantly more cytoplasm than is evident in lymphocytes, and the cytoplasm is rich in lysosomes containing various hydrolases.

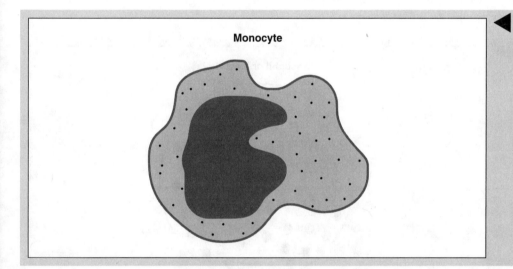
Monocyte

FIGURE 3-7
Monocyte or Macrophage. Both monocytes and macrophages are characterized by their irregular shape and a significant number of cytoplasmic granules. The cells have multiple roles in the immune response, including: (1) presenting antigens to the T lymphocytes, (2) producing monokines that help in the initiation and coordination of the immune response, and (3) working with the acquired immune system and complement to phagocytose and kill antibody or C3b-coated particles. Generally, an increased level of blood monocytes is an indication of the presence of a chronic immune response.

The monocyte and macrophage populations have multiple functions that are critical to a successful immune response. One set of functions is related to phagocytic ability. The cells routinely sample the environment by engulfing cells, particles, and macromolecules. Because the macrophage, in most cases, cannot distinguish between self- and nonself-structures, it samples everything in the environment and displays environmental antigens, both self- and nonself-structures, on its surface. T lymphocytes are necessary to make the distinction between foreign and self-structures. This process is called *antigen presentation*, and the monocytes and macrophages that perform this function are called antigen-presenting cells (APCs). Antigen presentation requires a unique cell-surface, antigen-holding structure called the class II major histocompatibility complex (MHC) molecule, which is essential for the successful initiation of acquired immune responses.

A second function of macrophages is to aid in the initiation and coordination of the immune response. In this capacity, the monocyte can be considered a chemical factory. It makes a variety of protein molecules called monokines, which play a central role in many aspects of the immune response. These functions are discussed in more detail in Chap. 6.

Finally, the monocyte or macrophage population mediates effector activities of the acquired immune system. In this capacity, the monocyte or macrophage can kill and efficiently phagocytose particles that are coated with antibody or C3b of the complement system. Although there are relatively low numbers of monocytes represented in the CBC, the cell type is, nevertheless, a very abundant type found in all tissues. Once in a tissue, the monocyte remains in that tissue.

Basophils and Mast Cells

Basophils circulate in the blood. **Mast cells** are fixed in tissues.

Like the other leukocytes, both the basophils and mast cells are of bone marrow origin and are distinguished based on location. Basophils are found circulating in the blood, whereas mast cells are fixed in tissues. Although the cells look and function identically and both derive from the bone marrow, the exact relationship of these cells to each other has not been clearly established. Schematically illustrated in Fig. 3-8, basophils and mast cells are characterized by the deep blue of their cytoplasmic granules following staining with the Wright's stain. The granules contain histamine and other preformed mediators of anaphylaxis. Both cell types also contain the metabolic machinery to produce a variety of lipid mediators (e.g., prostaglandins, leukotrienes) that can enhance and extend anaphylatic responses. Mast cells and basophils both express two unique cell-surface structures that are central to their function. One of these cell-surface structures is a receptor for the IgE molecule, which functions in allergic and anaphylactic reactions. The second cell-surface structure is a receptor for anaphylatoxin signals received from complement activation.

FIGURE 3-8

Basophil or Mast Cell. Both basophils and mast cells are characterized by a multi-lobed nucleus; abundant, large cytoplasmic granules; and a unique affinity for basic dyes. The two cell types are distinguished from each other by their location. Basophils are found in the circulation, and mast cells reside in the tissues. Both cells initiate inflammation (anaphylaxis) upon stimulation by antigen and IgE or by the activation of complement through the C3a component.

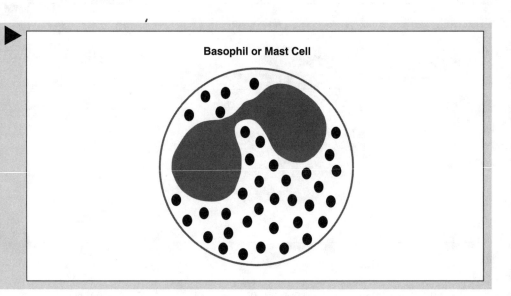

Basophil or Mast Cell

The function of basophils and mast cells can best be compared to that of a sentry. When antigen binds and cross-links cell-bound IgE or when C3a is being generated by activation of the complement cascade, the basophil or mast cell is triggered to degranulate, releasing histamine and other mediators of anaphylaxis. These mediators start the inflammatory reaction that allows components of the immune system to enter the area.

Eosinophils

Like neutrophils, the eosinophils are also phagocytic cells and are characterized by a multilobed nuclear structure (Fig. 3-9). In contrast to neutrophils, however, they have characteristic deep-red, eosin-staining cytoplasmic granules, indicating a major difference in the granule contents. Eosinophils are brought to the site of mast cell degranulation by a potent eosinophil chemotactic factor that is produced late in the mast cell degranulation response. The granules of the eosinophils contain histaminase and aryl-sulfatase, which can inactivate products of degranulated mast cells. Therefore, one function for these cells can be thought of as suppressing the reactions initiated by mast cell degranulation. A second proposed function for the eosinophils relates to the toxic activity that the major basic protein component of the eosinophil granule has on hel-

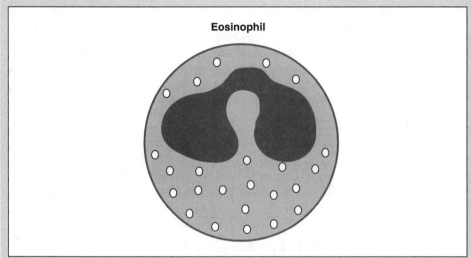

Eosinophil

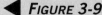

FIGURE 3-9
Eosinophil. *Eosinophils are granule-containing cells with multilobed nuclei that are characterized by their affinity for the dye eosin. The granules contain histaminase, which can potentially dampen or suppress the inflammation associated with mast-cell degranulation. In addition, a toxic major basic protein found in the eosinophil granules possesses a potent antihelminth activity along with a generalized cytotoxicity for several other cell types. An elevated eosinophil level usually indicates either an allergic response or infection with a helminth.*

minths. Eosinophils also express a cell-surface receptor for the carboxyl terminal, the Fc portion, of the antibody molecule, which allows the eosinophil to bind to antibody-coated parasites, releasing their major basic protein and killing the infecting organisms.

ORGANIZED LYMPHOID TISSUES

The leukocytes comprise only part of the immunologic anatomy that was responding to Sarah's infection. In Sarah's neck, the physician felt swollen, hard lymph nodes. Throughout the body there are similar aggregations of lymphoid tissues that include not only lymph nodes but also the spleen, bone marrow, and thymus, and other less well-defined lymphoid aggregates. The extent of the lymphoid tissues is illustrated in Fig. 3-10. This is clearly an oversimplification of the anatomy of the immune system, but it emphasizes the concept that components of the immune system are in intimate contact with all other tissues and organs. It is often simplest to consider lymphoid tissues in two basic categories based on function. These two categories are the central and the peripheral lymphoid tissues.

Central Lymphoid Tissues (Antigen-Independent Events)

The central lymphoid tissues include the bone marrow and the thymus gland. These are the tissues where the immune system develops. Lymphopoiesis, discussed in the beginning of this chapter, occurs primarily in the bone marrow. Whereas B lymphocytes start and complete their development in the bone marrow, T lymphocytes migrate from the bone marrow and complete their differentiation in the thymus. The developmental processes that occur in the central lymphoid tissues are preprogrammed and happen in the absence of antigen. During development in the central lymphoid tissues, each T and B lymphocyte generates its specific antigen-binding receptor. In other words, the ability to respond to a specific antigen is developed prior to exposure to the antigen. One can conceive of this process as the random development of a B- and T-lymphocyte library, with each cell in the library specific for an as yet unencountered antigen. The random nature of lymphocyte antigen-receptor development would be expected to generate cells capable of reacting with autologous molecules. To compensate for the generation of self-reacting lymphocytes, the newly generated cells must be "educated" not to react with self-tissues. Because of the differences in antigens for both the B and T lymphocytes, this process of education must be unique to each class of cells. The result of the process is regulation of lymphocyte responsiveness and tolerance for self-structures. If later in life this regulation or tolerance is broken, then the immune system is free to begin reacting with autologous structures, which gives rise to autoimmune disease.

FIGURE 3-10 ▶
Anatomy of the Immune System. This figure provides an overview of the immune system anatomy. The macroscopic anatomy consists of the central lymphoid tissues of the bone marrow and thymus and the peripheral lymphoid tissues of the lymph nodes, spleen, and other lymphoid aggregates. The microscopic anatomy is more complex in that lymphocytes and macrophages are found in all cells and tissues. The lymphocytes are mobile and circulate between the tissues and the lymphoid organs. Part of this circulation includes lymphatic vessels that channel circulation cells to the nodes.

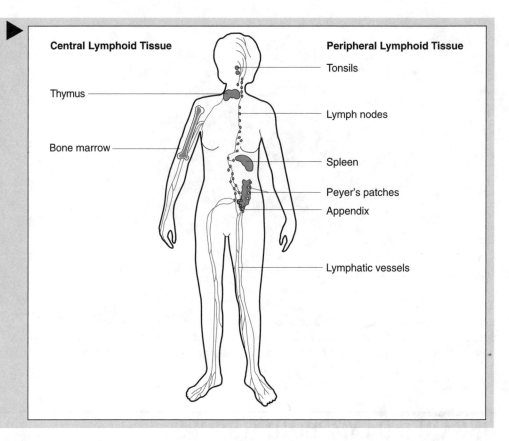

Central Lymphoid Tissue   **Peripheral Lymphoid Tissue**

Thymus

Bone marrow

Tonsils

Lymph nodes

Spleen

Peyer's patches

Appendix

Lymphatic vessels

Lymph Node Functional Areas
Afferent vessels
Paracortex
Cortex
Medulla
Efferent lymphatics

Peripheral Lymphoid Tissues (Antigen-Dependent Events)

Whereas antigen-independent events occur in the central lymphoid tissues, antigen-dependent events happen in the peripheral lymphoid tissues. The peripheral tissues consist of the lymphatic vessels, lymph nodes, and spleen as well as other aggregations of lymphocytes. Lymphoid aggregates are especially evident in mucosal tissues and include structures such as Peyer's patches, the tonsils, and the appendix.

Lymph Node. Fig. 3-10 indicates several cellular aggregations in the lymphatic circulation. The aggregations are called lymph nodes, and they are not a random collection of lymphocytes but rather an organization of cells that efficiently allow the required cells to interact and initiate an immune response. The structure of a typical lymph node is schematically illustrated in Fig. 3-11. The node consists of a capsule, where several afferent lymphatic vessels enter. Underneath the capsule is the cortex of the node, which is rich in B lymphocytes and contains primary and secondary lymphoid follicles. In the middle of the node is the medulla, an area rich in antibody-secreting plasma cells, and between the cortex and the medulla is the paracortical region. The paracortex is rich in APCs and T lymphocytes. Generally, the antigen or circulating lymphocytes enter the node from the afferent vessels. Cells and antigen leave the lymphatic vessels and are filtered through the paracortical region of the node, where they initially encounter antigen-presenting dendritic macrophages and T lymphocytes. Antigen flow is also directed to the B lymphocytes in the cortex. The design of this tissue provides maximum opportunity for antigen to encounter both B and T lymphocytes and for the B and T lymphocytes to interact with each other. In the primary follicular area of the node, a B lymphocyte that is stimulated by antigen and receives T-cell help begins to proliferate, and, in a relatively short period, undergoes in excess of 10 cell divisions. The newly synthesized cells must displace other resident cells and, in the process, create a secondary follicle. The progeny of the initially stimulated B lymphocyte continue their proliferation and differentiation in the germinal center of the newly created secondary follicle. Eventually, these cells leave the germinal center and complete their differentiation into either antibody-secreting plasma cells or long-lived memory cells. Antigen stimulation of

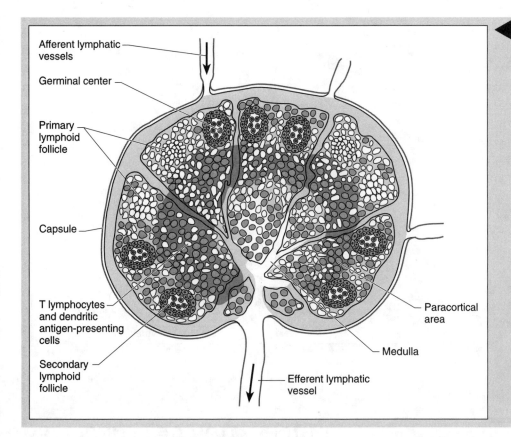

Afferent lymphatic vessels

Germinal center

Primary lymphoid follicle

Capsule

T lymphocytes and dendritic antigen-presenting cells

Secondary lymphoid follicle

Paracortical area

Medulla

Efferent lymphatic vessel

◀ **FIGURE 3-11**
Structure of the Lymph Node. *Antigen or circulating lymphocytes enter the lymph node through the afferent lymphatic vessels. In the cortical area of the node are aggregations of B cells called the primary lymphoid follicles. When a B cell in a primary follicle begins proliferating, the follicle takes on the structure of a secondary follicle, with a ring of B lymphocytes around the developing plasma cells and memory in the germinal center of the follicle. The paracortical area of the node is rich in T lymphocytes and antigen-presenting macrophages called dendritic cells. It is in the paracortical area of the node that T-lymphocyte stimulation takes place. Mature plasma cells that secrete antibody molecules are located in the medulla of the node. The secreted antibodies and lymphocytes leave the node through the efferent lymphatic vessels.*

B and T lymphocytes need not take place in the same individual lymph node. For example, the developing daughter cell of an antigen-stimulated T cell may encounter the corresponding antigen-stimulated B cell in a different node altogether.

Spleen. One function of the spleen is the removal of old or misshapen RBCs, which occurs in an area of the spleen called the red pulp. A second splenic function, however, takes place in the spleen's white pulp. This second function is a filtering of antigen, which is analogous to the filtering taking place in the lymph node. Fig. 3-12 illustrates the functional organization of the lymphoid components of the spleen. In contrast to the lymph node, which filters and detects antigen in the lymphatics, the spleen filters and detects antigen in the blood. Blood-borne antigen enters the spleen through the splenic artery. As the antigens leave the circulation, they encounter a sheath of lymphocytes surrounding the artery. This periarterial sheath of lymphocytes is rich in APCs and T lymphocytes. In a process identical to that of the lymph node, the antigens progress to the follicular area of the spleen, where B lymphocytes are clonally selected and receive help from the selected T cells. These cells then proliferate and eventually differentiate into either plasma or memory cells. Analogous to the events in the lymph nodes, lymphocyte proliferation and differentiation start in primary splenic follicles and result in the generation of secondary splenic follicles. In both the nodes and the spleen and in the presence of a large antigen load, the elevated level of B-cell stimulation and proliferation leads to the development of several germinal centers. As a result, the entire structure, lymph node or spleen, can enlarge (as did the lymph nodes in Sarah's neck). Organisms or fragments of organisms colonizing in Sarah's throat have broken through the innate immune defenses of her skin and mucosal membranes and were trapped in her local lymph nodes. The cells in these nodes are now responding to those antigens.

Other Lymphatic Structures. Lymphoid aggregations and the formation of germinal centers are not limited to the lymph nodes and spleen. Several other tissues, especially tissues of the gastrointestinal tract and mucosal tissues, exhibit similar structures. Examples of the other organized lymphatic structures include Peyer's patches and the tonsils.

FIGURE 3-12 ▶

Structure of the Spleen. *The functional structure of the spleen is similar to that of the lymph node. In this case, blood antigens and lymphocytes leave the splenic arteries and encounter a periarterial sheath of T lymphocytes and antigen-presenting cells. B cells are found in primary follicles, and when a B cell is activated, the proliferating cells develop a secondary follicle.*

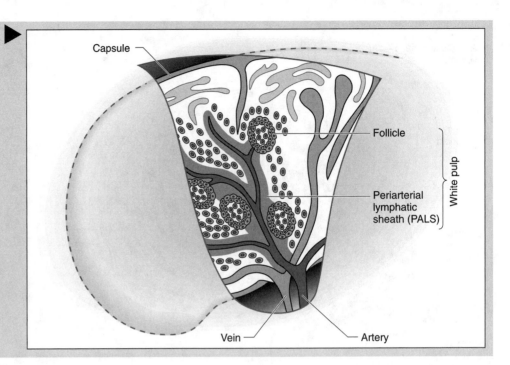

CIRCULATION OF LEUKOCYTES

By this point, it should be clear that the immune system can best be considered as a liquid organ system. Like all organ systems, the leukocyte populations consist of different cells that communicate with each other to carry out their required functions. The leukocytes, however, are individual cells that can move from one site to another within their organ system. Different leukocyte populations, however, have different migratory patterns.

Circulation of Neutrophils and Monocytes

Like all of the leukocytes, the neutrophils and monocytes are synthesized in the bone marrow from the pluripotent stem cell. Upon maturation, these cells leave the marrow, and migrate through the blood, and when signaled by an inflammatory event, they leave the blood and enter the tissues. This is a one-way trip during which the cells either remain in the tissue or are activated in the tissue by the inflammatory event, perform their functions, and eventually die. The lifetime of the neutrophils is relatively short, requiring the bone marrow to synthesize billions of cells every day. Tissue macrophages, on the other hand, may have a significantly longer lifetime. However, once they have entered a tissue, macrophages remain in that tissue.

Lymphatic Circulation

Like monocytes and neutrophils, lymphocytes are also generated in the bone marrow and leave the marrow. However, unlike the other leukocytes, lymphocytes have the capability to enter and leave the tissues. As a result, lymphocytes circulate between tissues, nodes, spleen, and blood.

Antigens and cells contained within the interstitial fluid space or blood are in contact with the peripheral lymphoid organs via the lymphatic circulation. This circulatory system is also illustrated in Fig. 3-10, which depicts how either antigen or a lymphocyte in an interstitial space can be directed to one of the lymph nodes. The lymphatic fluid is in a continuous one-way flow from the tissues to the nodes and finally empties into the venous circulatory system at the thoracic duct. The flow of the lymphatic cells and antigens in the interstitial fluid is maintained by normal muscular contractions and body movement. The unidirectionality of the flow, directing the fluid to a lymph node, is maintained by small valves present in the lymphatic vessels.

RESOLUTION OF CLINICAL CASE

All of these cells worked together in Sarah to help fight her streptococcal infection. Colonization by the infecting organism damages tissues, which activates the inflammatory response. Signal molecules released by the inflammation allow neutrophils to leave the blood and enter the area of inflammation. Bacteria and bacterial products that are in the interstitial fluid are directed to the local lymph nodes, where B and T lymphocytes are activated. The large antigen load activates several B and T lymphocytes, resulting in the development of several new germinal centers and causing the node to enlarge, which was detected by Sarah's physician. Maturing lymphocytes leave the node and take up residence in other nodes or tissues to prepare for any specific antigen entering other tissues. Some of the activated B lymphocytes enter the medullary area of the node and complete their differentiation into plasma cells that secrete antibody, whereas other activated B lymphocytes complete their maturation in different locations. Antibody synthesized by plasma cells leaves the node and eventually enters the circulation, where it is in equilibrium with the interstitial fluids. The antibody can then bind to the infecting streptococcal organisms and help in the elimination of the infection by interacting with many of the other leukocyte populations that have entered the infected tissue. The method by which antigen stimulates the B and T lymphocytes is the subject of Chap. 4.

REVIEW QUESTIONS

Directions: For each of the following questions, choose the **one best** answer.

1. The following white blood cell count (WBC) is most consistent with which one of the following conditions?

	Patient	*Normal Values*
WBC count	$10 \times 10^3/\mu L$	$7–14 \times 10^3/\mu L$
Segmented neutrophils	62%	60%–70%
Banded neutrophils	0%	0%–5%
Lymphocytes	25%	20%–40%
Monocytes	5%	2%–6%
Basophils	0%	0%–1%
Eosinophils	8%	1%–4%

   (A) Bacterial infection
   (B) Viral infection
   (C) Tissue necrosis
   (D) Allergic reaction
   (E) Chronic infection

2. Which of the following functions is associated primarily with the neutrophils?
   (A) Acute response to bacteria and necrotic tissue
   (B) Chronic inflammatory responses
   (C) Responses to viral infections
   (D) Distinguishing between self- and nonself-antigens
   (E) Initiating anaphylactic reactions

3. In which area of the lymph node is one most likely to detect macrophages presenting antigen to T lymphocytes?
   (A) Subcapsular space
   (B) Cortex
   (C) Paracortex
   (D) Medulla
   (E) Primary lymphoid follicle

4. Which one of the following events is unique to the central lymphoid tissues?
   (A) Interaction of antigen with B lymphocytes
   (B) Interaction between T lymphocytes and B lymphocytes
   (C) Degranulation of mast cells
   (D) Differentiation of B lymphocytes into plasma cells
   (E) Differentiation of a stem cell into a lymphoid progenitor cell

5. Which one of the following cell types carries a memory of previously encountered antigen?
  (A) Neutrophils
  (B) Lymphocytes
  (C) Monocytes
  (D) Basophils
  (E) Eosinophils

6. Which one of the following cell types is responsible for the antigen specificity of the immune response?
  (A) Neutrophils
  (B) Lymphocytes
  (C) Monocytes
  (D) Basophils
  (E) Eosinophils

7. Mast cells and basophils differ from each other in which one of the following characteristics?
  (A) The inflammatory mediators found in their granules
  (B) The immunologic reactions in which they participate
  (C) Their location
  (D) Their ability to synthesize lipid mediators

8. All of the cells that make up the immune system are derived from which single cell type?
  (A) Fibroblasts
  (B) Epithelial cells
  (C) Lymphocytes
  (D) Bone marrow stem cells

9. A complete blood count that indicates an elevated number of banded neutrophils would be most consistent with which one of the following conditions?
  (A) An early response to viral infection
  (B) Acute viral infection
  (C) Chronic bacterial infection
  (D) Acute bacterial infection
  (E) Fungal infection

10. The central and peripheral lymphoid tissues differ from each other in which one of the following characteristics?
  (A) B cells are found in the central lymphoid tissue, and T cells are found in the peripheral tissues.
  (B) The central and peripheral lymphoid tissues have identical functions but are found in different locations.
  (C) Antigen plays a role in the central lymphoid tissues but not in the peripheral lymphoid tissues.
  (D) Antigen plays a role in the peripheral lymphoid tissues but not in the central lymphoid tissues.

ANSWERS AND EXPLANATIONS

1. **The answer is D.** During the course of an allergic reaction, the mast cell releases multiple mediators. The granule contents of mast cells contain histamine and other mediators, which are responsible for most of the immediate inflammatory activity. The degranulated mast cell also synthesizes many other products that augment and modify the initial inflammation. One of these mediators stimulates and is chemotactic for eosinophils. Chronic mast-cell degranulation is then associated with elevations in eosinophils. Infections with helminths also increase eosinophil levels.

2. **The answer is A.** Neutrophils are primarily thought of as a necessary component for killing bacteria and responding to necrotic tissues. Neutrophils are usually considered as part of the first or acute response to any infection. As the response to the infection becomes chronic in nature, lymphocytes and macrophages predominantly respond.

3. **The answer is C.** One of the first areas that an antigen traverses on its path through the lymph node is the paracortical area, where dendritic macrophages present antigens to T lymphocytes. The cortex is rich in B lymphocytes that can also bind antigen. Once the B lymphocytes bind antigen and receive T-cell help, the B lymphocytes begin proliferating and differentiating, forming the secondary lymphoid follicle. In the medulla, plasma cells are synthesizing antibody.

4. **The answer is E.** The central lymphoid tissues, bone marrow, and thymus are the sites of the development of the immune system and are antigen free or antigen independent (unless there is an infection of these tissues). The other options listed are events that take place in response to antigens and are termed antigen-dependent events.

5. **The answer is B.** Whereas all of the cell types can interact with antibody specifically to remove or kill the target antigen, none of the cells by themselves have the capability of carrying the memory of an immune reaction, except the lymphocytes.

6. **The answer is B.** Lymphocytes also provide the specificity of immunologic reactions. On their cell surface, B cells and T cells carry specific receptors for antigen. In comparing two B cells, the cell structures and functions are identical except for the limited portion of the antigen receptor that binds antigen. A similar pattern is observed for T cells. None of the other choices in this question have an antigen-specific reactivity and must rely on antibody to direct their function specifically to target cells.

7. **The answer is C.** The functions of these two cell types are identical. Mast cells are found in the tissues, and basophils are found in the circulation. The developmental relationship between these two cell types is, however, unclear.

8. **The answer is D.** The hematopoietic system is totally dependent on the bone marrow stem cell type. Under the influence of the appropriate growth and differentiation factors, the stem cell gives rise to all components of the hematopoietic system.

9. **The answer is C.** During a bacterial infection, the bone marrow is stimulated to release neutrophils. If the signal persists, immature neutrophils (banded neutrophils) are also released. The longer the stimulus persists, the greater the number of immature cells seen in the circulation.

10. **The answer is D.** Lymphocyte development and education takes place in the central lymphoid tissues in the absence of antigen.

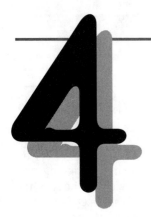

ACTIVATION OF THE IMMUNE RESPONSE

INTRODUCTION OF CLINICAL CASE

Jane Czerwinski, a 15-month-old infant, was brought to the family practice clinic for her routine well-child examination. During the course of her office visit, Jane received her first measles immunization.

ACTIVATION OF ACQUIRED IMMUNE SYSTEM

During Jane's visit to her family physician, she was exposed to an attenuated measles virus. This immunization required Jane's immune system to respond to an organism that she had never previously encountered. As a result of this response, Jane needs to develop antibody to the measles virus. To accomplish this, an appropriate B lymphocyte that has the capability of producing an antibody that specifically binds the virus must be selected. This is called B-cell clonal selection. In addition, cytotoxic T lymphocytes that can recognize and kill virus-infected cells also must be selected. This is called T-cell clonal selection. The cells in Jane that were selected by the measles virus are specific for that virus and would not be selected by another unrelated virus.

CLONAL SELECTION OF B LYMPHOCYTES

Development of the B-Lymphocyte Antigen Receptor

Isotypes and Idiotypes
The term isotype refers to the type or class of antibody. The term idiotype refers to the unique characteristics of the portion of the antibody molecule or cell receptor that directly binds antigen.

The previous chapter discussed the characteristics and cell-surface markers of B lymphocytes. One of the surface structures on B cells that is central to understanding their function is the B-cell receptor for antigen. This antigen receptor is an antibody of the immunoglobulin M (IgM) isotype. The antigen-binding specificity of the B-cell receptor is established during normal B-cell development. Individual B cells then differ from each other only in the unique characteristics of their antigen-binding site; that is, each B cell that develops in the bone marrow has its own unique antigen-binding identity. The term *idiotype* is used to refer to this unique antigen-binding site. For example, two different B lymphocytes that bind different antigens would have different idiotypes, although both antigen-binding molecules are of the IgM isotype. On the other hand, if an IgM and an IgG antibody both contained the identical antigen-binding site, then these two different isotype antibodies would share a common idiotype. IgM, IgG, IgE, and IgA are all different isotypes.

Fig. 4-1 schematically illustrates the process of B-lymphocyte ontogeny. When the lymphoid progenitor cell receives the information that commits it to the B-lymphocyte lineage, a series of antigen-independent events starts taking place. In one of the first events, the gene that codes for the immunoglobulin molecule is rearranged. This rearrangement process involves randomly selecting individual gene fragments, which are necessary to construct the deoxyribonucleic acid (DNA) that will eventually code for the antigen-binding site of the B cell's membrane IgM. Therefore, antigen-binding specificity develops before the individual ever encounters antigen. Once the developing B lymphocyte produces a successful rearrangement of the immunoglobulin gene, the enzymes necessary for the rearrangement processes are inactivated. As a result, each B lymphocyte is able to produce a unique IgM molecule with one unique antigen-binding site. This unique antigen-binding site defines the B cell's idiotype. All antibody molecules produced by a single B cell have the identical antigen-binding specificity, that is, the identical idiotype. The progeny of that original B cell will all express the identical IgM molecule with the identical antigen-binding specificity. These daughter cells are clones of the original cell.

Following the initial rearrangement of the immunoglobulin gene, differentiation continues with the synthesis of the IgM polypeptide chains, the assembly of the IgM

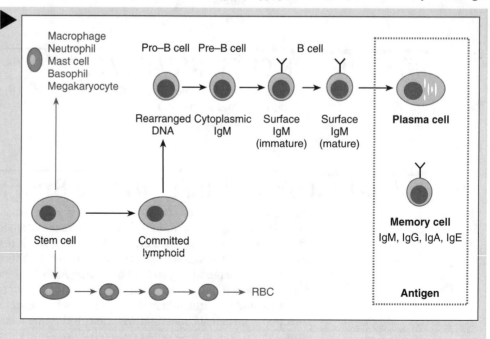

FIGURE 4-1

B-Lymphocyte Ontogeny. *B lymphocytes develop in the bone marrow from a pluripotent stem cell. The developmental process follows a logical progression of events in which, initially, the DNA that will eventually code for the antibody molecule is rearranged. This apparently random rearrangement generates a gene fragment that will code for the antigen-combining site of the antibody molecule. Once a successful rearrangement occurs, no future rearrangements are permitted, so that one cell makes antibody with only one binding specificity. Following the DNA rearrangement process, the heavy and light polypeptide chains of the IgM molecule are synthesized and assembled. The completed molecule is then expressed on the surface of the B lymphocyte. This entire process happens in the absence of antigen. In the presence of antigen, a mature B cell can be clonally selected and complete the process by differentiating into either a plasma cell or a memory cell.*

molecule, and the incorporation of the IgM molecule into the cell membrane. These developing cells eventually mature into the B lymphocytes. The peripheral B-cell population can then be considered as a library of cells. However, each cell in the library is capable of selectively binding different antigens.

In Jane's case, the measles virus vaccine can bind only to the antigen-binding site on a select subset of B cells, with an affinity for the antigen. Illustrated in Fig. 4-2, this process is clonal selection.

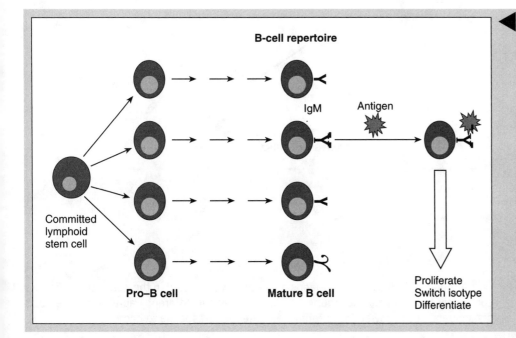

B-cell repertoire

IgM   Antigen

Committed
lymphoid
stem cell

Proliferate
Switch isotype
Differentiate

Pro–B cell   **Mature B cell**

FIGURE 4-2
Clonal Selection of B Lymphocytes. *B-cell ontogeny results in the generation of a library of B lymphocytes all expressing IgM molecules on the cell surface with a different antigen-binding site. In the presence of antigen, the antigen will bind to the B cells in the library with an antibody-combining site capable of holding the antigen. These selected cells are stimulated (promoted to the G_1 phase [resting phase] of the cell cycle from a noncycling, or G_O, cell). To mount a successful immune response, the selected cell must proliferate, switch from the IgM isotype to an antibody isotype more appropriate to the stimulating antigen, and differentiate into either a plasma cell or a memory cell. The information to accomplish differentiation comes from helper T lymphocytes.*

Upon clonal selection of the B cell by antigen, the B cell is activated and poised to carry out its immunologic function. The eventual fate of this activated B cell, however, depends on several factors related to both the nature of the antigen and the immunologic situation of the host. To mount an antibody response successfully, selected B lymphocytes need to proliferate, producing large numbers of daughter cells with identical antigen-binding specificity. The B lymphocyte must also change the isotype of antibody that it can produce to respond most effectively to the infecting antigen. Finally, the B lymphocyte must eventually differentiate into a plasma cell that can produce and secrete antibody molecules or into a memory B cell that can retain the ability to respond rapidly should the system encounter the antigen a second time. Success in these two activities depends on the nature of the antigen and the availability of help from T lymphocytes.

Clonally selected B lymphocytes must:
• Proliferate
• Switch isotypes
• Differentiate into either memory cells or plasma cells

T-Independent B-Cell Antigens

One type of antigen that can clonally select B lymphocytes is called a T-independent antigen. These antigens are usually polymers of an identical repeating structure. Because all antibodies on the cell surface have the identical binding site for antigen and because the T-independent antigens have a repeating identical structure, these antigens can cross-link several of the B cell's surface immunoglobulin molecules. Cross-linking alters IgM synthesis at the RNA level, and instead of producing a membrane-bound form of the antibody, a pentameric molecule is produced, which is secreted. When antigen no longer cross-links the cell-surface IgM receptor, the cell's metabolism reverts to making the membrane-bound form of the antibody. This T-independent activation of B lymphocytes is schematically illustrated in Fig. 4-3. The T-independent responses are rapid; however, there is no immunologic memory or isotype switching associated with the T-independent response.

T-Independent Response
This is a rapid IgM response to antigens with repeating polymeric structures, such as bacteria. There is no isotype switch and no memory.

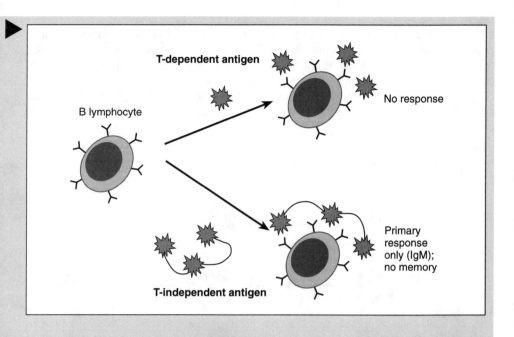

FIGURE 4-3
T-Dependent and T-Independent Antigens. Two different types of antigens select B lymphocytes: T-dependent and T-independent antigens. Most antigens are T-dependent and require help from T cells to proliferate, switch isotypes, and differentiate into either plasma cells or memory cells. All immune responses that generate immunologic memory are T-dependent responses. T-independent antigens have a unique structure. These antigens are represented by polymers of repeating structure, such as bacterial cell walls. The polymeric material can bind to and cross-link the IgM molecules on the B-cell's surface. This event alters the protein synthetic machinery of the B lymphocyte, and instead of synthesizing a membrane-bound IgM molecule, the cell synthesizes and secretes a pentameric IgM molecule. This is an important response to some bacteria because it happens rapidly; however, no isotype switching is involved in the response, and there is no immunologic memory of previous encounters with identical bacteria.

Although T-independent antigens are relatively restricted in their structure, they are commonly found in the polymeric cell wall of several different bacterial species and consequently can play an important role in the rapid response to bacteria.

T-Dependent B-Cell Antigens

T-Dependent Response
This is the response to most antigens that, with the help of T lymphocytes, allows the immune system to develop a memory of the initial antigen exposure and produce antibodies of the IgG, IgE, and IgA isotypes.

The second major classification of B-cell antigens is that of a T-dependent antigen. The term T-dependent refers to the need for T lymphocytes to provide the information necessary to allow clonally selected B lymphocytes to proliferate, switch isotypes, and differentiate. Until Jane is able to initiate a T-lymphocyte response successfully, she will not succeed in producing an effective antibody response to the measles vaccine.

CLONAL SELECTION OF T LYMPHOCYTES

T lymphocytes and B lymphocytes are functionally identical in one very important characteristic: both have the capability to react with a specific antigen. Both the B lymphocyte and T lymphocyte provide the acquired immune response, with its unique characteristic of antigen specificity and immunologic memory. However, T lymphocytes and B lymphocytes differ in the type of antigen receptor displayed on the cell surface, that is, in the nature of the antigen that stimulates the different cells and in the eventual function of the clonally selected lymphocytes.

T-Lymphocyte Antigens

B-lymphocyte antigens *bind directly to the IgM B-cell antigen receptor.*
T-lymphocyte antigens *must be processed to allow them to be held on the surface of the host's cells.*

Like the B cell, the T lymphocyte has a cell-surface structure that is capable of specifically binding antigen. The development of the T-cell antigen receptor (TCR) starts in the bone marrow and is analogous to that already described for the B lymphocyte. The end product of this developmental pathway is the random generation of a set of T lymphocytes, each of which can display TCR for different antigens. Using mechanisms analogous to B lymphocytes, each individual T lymphocyte expresses TCRs with a unique binding specificity. These T lymphocytes are then available for clonal selection by antigen.

Antigens that select T lymphocytes are different from antigens that select B lymphocytes. B-lymphocyte antigens bind directly to the antigen-combining site on the B-cell

IgM receptor. T-lymphocyte antigens, on the other hand, must be displayed on the surface of another host cell. This limitation of requiring all T-cell antigens to be displayed on a membrane could be overcome by one all-encompassing binding molecule. This would require all of the host's cells to have structures on the exterior of their cell membranes, which are capable of binding and displaying all possible antigens that the cell might either encounter (virus) or make (mutated protein). A single molecule with all the specificity and range of binding activities of the entire immune system does not exist. The alternate approach to this problem (the approach used by the immune system) is to chemically change or process T-cell antigens to increase the probability that they will be held by a set of common antigen-holding structures.

Antigen Processing

The process of converting T-lymphocyte antigens into structures that can be displayed on a cell's surface is called antigen processing. There are two different antigen-processing pathways and, not unexpectedly, two different groups of cell-surface structures to hold the processed antigen. There are also two different types of T lymphocytes that are clonally selected by these pathways. These different pathways are often classified by the nature of the cell-surface structure that eventually holds the processed antigen.

Major Histocompatibility Complex

The cell-surface structures that are responsible for displaying antigens are included in the group of molecules collectively referred to as the major histocompatibility complex (MHC) antigens or the human leukocyte antigens (HLA). Unfortunately, nomenclature is one of the major problems encountered in attempting to understand the structure and function of the MHC molecules.

The term *major histocompatibility complex* is a generic term that refers to this set of proteins in any species. *Human leukocyte antigen* refers to the MHC proteins in the human, while a different term is used to refer to the MHC proteins in other species. To complicate the issue even further, the MHC includes more proteins and functions than just the antigen-holding structures found on cell surfaces. This incredibly complex collection of proteins has major biologic functions in several growth and developmental processes. Fortunately, to understand the immune system, we only need to focus on two groups of MHC molecules. These groups of molecules are the class I MHC and class II MHC proteins. However, within each of the two large classes there are multiple individual proteins that differ from each other, primarily in the portion of the molecule that directly contacts the processed antigen. This heterogeneity in class I MHC– and class II MHC– binding sites is biologically important because it provides an increased possibility of holding all antigens that the host might encounter.

Although the polypeptide chains that constitute the class I and class II molecules are different, there is an extraordinary three-dimensional similarity between them. The major differences between class I MHC and class II MHC molecules are in tissue distribution, the antigen-processing pathway, and the types of T lymphocytes that can be selected by each of the classes (Table 4-1).

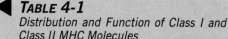

TABLE 4-1
Distribution and Function of Class I and Class II MHC Molecules

	Class I MHC	Class II MHC
Different molecules within the class	HLA-A HLA-B HLA-C	HLA-DP HLA-DQ HLA-DR
Location	All nucleated cells	Antigen-presenting cells, B cells, and activated T cells (lower concentrations on some other cell types)
Antigen source	Synthesized within the cell	Extracellular
Antigen presented to	Cytotoxic T cells (CD8)	Helper T cells (CD4)

Note. HLA = human leukocyte antigen. Letters following HLA designate genetic loci.

ANTIGEN-PROCESSING PATHWAYS

As suggested above, there are two different antigen-processing pathways, and the pathway used depends on where the antigen was synthesized.

Class I MHC Processing

If the antigen is synthesized within the cell, then the newly synthesized antigen is processed by the pathway illustrated in Fig. 4-4. In this pathway, synthesized antigen is directed to a cytoplasmic proteasome, where it is proteolytically fragmented. The resulting fragments are then targeted to an endosomal compartment of the cell containing class I MHC molecules. The antigen fragments then have an opportunity to bind to the class I MHC molecule. The endosomal structure, containing class I MHC-bound–antigen fragments, migrates to and fuses with the cell membrane, resulting in the cell-surface display of the class I MHC–antigen complex. Antigen fragments that do not bind to the complex are not retained on the surface and are no longer involved in the immune response. All synthesized antigens are involved in this process, including normal self-proteins, mutated self-proteins, and foreign structures, such as the virus that is infecting Jane's cells. All nucleated cells, then, constantly display processed products of their synthetic apparatus on the cell surface. It is the role of the cytotoxic T lymphocyte (CD8 cell) to discriminate between the products that belong and those that should be removed.

> **Class I MHC Processing**
> - Antigen is synthesized within the presenting cell.
> - The pathway is active in all nucleated cells.
> - Antigen is presented to CD8 cytotoxic T lymphocytes.

FIGURE 4-4 ▶

Class I MHC Processing Pathway. *A sample of antigen synthesized within a cell is targeted to a cytoplasmic proteasome structure by the ubiquitin system. The newly synthesized protein is then fragmented by the proteasome, and the fragments are delivered to an endosome containing class I MHC molecules. Antigen fragments are allowed to bind to the class I MHC molecule, and the entire complex is directed to the cell surface, where the antigen fragments are presented to the CD8 cytotoxic T lymphocytes. Any antigen fragments that cannot bind to the class I MHC molecule will not be able to select CD8 lymphocytes.*

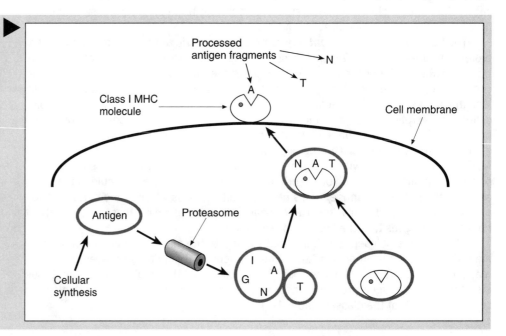

Class II MHC Processing

If the antigen is synthesized outside of a host cell, such as a bacterial protein or an injected structure like a protein vaccine, then the extracellular material is processed using the pathway illustrated in Fig. 4-5. In this case, the processed antigen is displayed on class II MHC molecules. Because of the limited tissue distribution of the class II MHC molecules, not all nucleated cells have this pathway available to them. Cells involved in this processing pathway are B lymphocytes, activated T lymphocytes, and, importantly, the macrophages, monocytes, and the tissue histiocytes, which are referred to collectively as antigen-presenting cells (APCs). By definition, the term APC is used to refer to histiocytes that express class II MHC molecules. However, all nucleated cells can present

> An **APC** presents antigen on class II MHC molecules and clonally selects a CD4 helper T lymphocyte.

antigens on the class I MHC molecules and, in that capacity, function as an APC. To complicate the issue further, not all class II MHC–expressing cells are able to perform the functions necessary to select efficiently the CD4 T cells. The key characteristic of an APC then is the ability to present antigen on class II MHC molecules and effectively clonally select a CD4 helper T lymphocyte. To help distinguish these different types of antigen presentation, some immunologists refer to cells that effectively present antigen to CD4 helper T lymphocytes as "professional APCs."

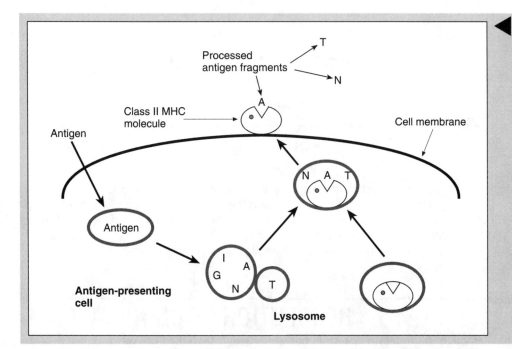

FIGURE 4-5
Class II MHC Processing Pathway. Extracellular antigen is engulfed by antigen-presenting cells, and the phagocytic vacuoles containing the antigen fuse with lysosomes. The antigen is then processed by the hydrolases of the lysosomes, and the resulting antigen fragments then fuse with an endosome containing the class II MHC molecule. Antigen fragments are allowed to bind to the class II MHC molecule, and the entire complex is directed to the cell surface, where the class II MHC–antigen complex is presented to CD4 helper T lymphocytes. Antigen fragments that cannot bind to the class II MHC molecule cannot select a helper T lymphocyte.

APCs sample molecules in the environment by phagocytosis. This sampling includes both normal host molecules, as well as antigenic material. The resulting phagosome then fuses with a lysosome, and the environmental molecules are digested by the lysosomal enzymes. This phagolysosome then combines with an endosome containing the class II MHC molecules, and the resulting macromolecular complex is directed to the cell membrane. This results in the cell-surface display of antigen fragments held by the class II MHC molecule. It is the role of the CD4 helper T cell to discriminate between products that belong and products that should be removed.

Development of T-Lymphocyte Antigen Receptor

The antigen structure that selects T lymphocytes is a combination of processed antigen peptide and a MHC molecule. The molecular complex, consisting of TCR, antigen fragment, and MHC molecule, is generally referred to as the *trimolecular complex*. This complex is schematically illustrated in Fig. 4-6. When the complex forms, the immune system can be activated. If something is done to interfere with the formation of this complex, there will be no immune response. If the MHC–antigen complex involves a class I MHC molecule, then a CD8 cytotoxic T lymphocyte is selected. If the MHC–antigen complex involves a class II MHC molecule, then a CD4 helper T lymphocyte is selected.

The mechanism described above for selection of T lymphocytes puts some new and different constraints on the TCR. Unlike B cells that bind antigen directly, the T lymphocytes must be able to recognize not only antigen but also the cell-surface class I or class II MHC molecules. Since the antigen-combining portion of TCRs are randomly constructed, it is reasonable to assume that some of the TCRs that are initially generated from the pluripotent stem cell will fail to bind an individual's own class I or class II molecules. This will result in a failure to interact with any MHC-bound antigen. The development of T cells, then, requires that the immature T lymphocytes go through an additional "educa-

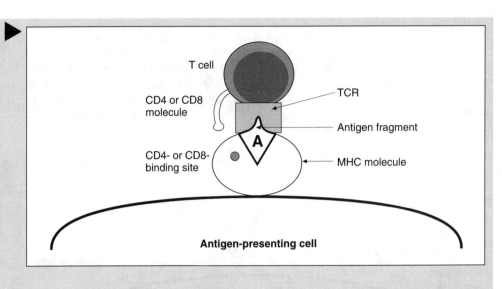

FIGURE 4-6
Clonal Selection of T Cells. The T-cell receptor for antigen binds a complex of both the antigen fragment and the MHC molecule. This complex containing the T-cell receptor (TCR), antigen fragment, and MHC molecule is referred to as the trimolecular complex. In addition, there is a binding site on the MHC molecule for either the CD4 or CD8 molecule. Class I MHC molecules have a binding site for the CD8 molecule, and class II MHC molecules have a binding site for the CD4 molecule. Clonal selection is a complex event that also includes interactions between several other T-cell and presenting cell-surface proteins. However, if either the antigen or the TCR that complements the antigen is missing, the T cell is not selected.

T cell

CD4 or CD8 molecule

TCR

Antigen fragment

CD4- or CD8-binding site

MHC molecule

A

Antigen-presenting cell

tion" process in which only the cells capable of binding MHC molecules will survive. In children, this education process happens in the thymus gland, one of the central lymphoid organs. This thymic dependency for T-cell function is the origin of the term *thymic-dependent lymphocyte*, or T lymphocyte. Fig. 4-7 presents a schematic illustration of T-lymphocyte ontogeny and the role of the thymus in T-cell development.

RESOLUTION OF CLINICAL CASE

Although the immune system is not well enough described, as yet, to know how the system protects Jane against a measles virus infection, it should be clear how B lymphocytes, CD4 helper T lymphocytes, and CD8 cytotoxic T lymphocytes can be activated by the patient's vaccination. The student should be able to follow the course of this vaccine as it selects cells of the immune system. Refer to Chap. 3 to identify in which anatomic location these events happen.

Fig. 4-8 illustrates the components of the immune system and outlines their rela-

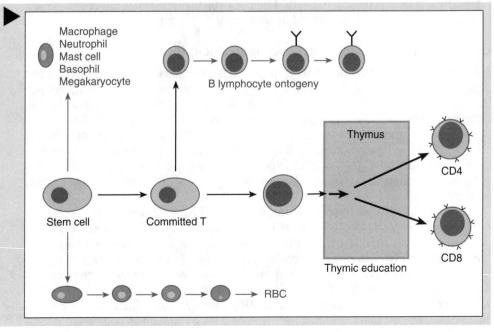

FIGURE 4-7
Thymic Education of T Lymphocytes. Like the B cells, T lymphocytes develop in the bone marrow. This development includes the random, antigen-independent development of the T-cell receptor (TCR). Partway through the developmental process, T cells leave the bone marrow and migrate to the thymus. In the thymus, T cells with TCRs that do not successfully bind to MHC molecules are eliminated. In addition, there may be cells present that bind to self-molecules and can generate autoimmune responses and cause disease. These cells are regulated to become tolerant of autoantigens. Mature CD4 and CD8 T lymphocytes leave the thymus.

Macrophage
Neutrophil
Mast cell
Basophil
Megakaryocyte

B lymphocyte ontogeny

Thymus

CD4

CD8

Stem cell

Committed T

Thymic education

RBC

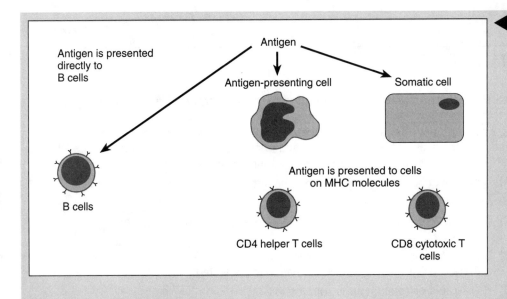

FIGURE 4-8
Overview of Clonal Selection. *The critical cells for antigen specificity and immunologic memory are the B and T lymphocytes. Intact antigen directly binds to and selects only the B cell that expresses a surface IgM molecule that complements the antigen. In most cases, this selected B cell needs help from CD4 helper T cells to continue the differentiation process and make antibody. T lymphocytes are selected differently by antigen. CD8 cytotoxic T lymphocytes are selected by antigen that has been synthesized within a cell and processed and presented on class I MHC molecules. All nucleated somatic cells can perform this function. Like the B cell, the selected CD8 cells need help from CD4 helper T cells to respond effectively to the antigen. Helper T cells are selected by extracellular antigen that has been engulfed by an antigen-presenting cell and presented on the class II MHC molecules. For a successful immune response, it is critical that the selected CD4 helper T cells proliferate and seed other sites, where the progeny of the initially selected cell can help either B or T lymphocytes perform their unique functions.*

tionship in the response to both intracellular and extracellular antigens. The methods for selecting B lymphocytes, helper T lymphocytes, and cytotoxic T lymphocytes are important fundamental immune reactions. Central to this process is the basic immunologic concept of clonal selection. How selected cells interact with each other both to remove antigen and to produce a memory of the response, in part, completes the missing portions of this figure.

REVIEW QUESTIONS

Directions: For each of the following questions, choose the **one best** answer.

1. A drug was developed that specifically prevents phagocytic vacuoles from being acidified. The enzymes in these structures require an acidic medium to function. What effect would this compound have on the immune response?

    (A) There would be no effect on the immune response.

    (B) APCs could not effectively present antigens to CD4 lymphocytes.

    (C) Nucleated cells could not effectively present antigens to CD8 cytotoxic T lymphocytes.

    (D) B-cell synthesis of all antibody isotypes would be normal because only the cell-mediated presentation would be adversely affected.

    (E) There would be total immune suppression.

2. Which of the following observations would be expected in a patient whose T cells failed to develop?

    (A) No antibody would be synthesized.

    (B) The antibody response would be normal because the T cells are affected but not the B cells.

    (C) The serum would contain normal to elevated levels of IgM antibody.

    (D) Only cell-mediated immunologic responses would be absent.

3. Which of the following is a consequence of thymic education of T lymphocytes?

    (A) Antigen-binding diversity of T cells is generated.

    (B) Antigen-binding diversity of B cells is generated.

    (C) An antigen presented on a nonhost MHC molecule will not react with T cells that were clonally selected by the identical antigen presented in the host.

    (D) The TCR is developed.

4. B and T lymphocytes differ from each other in which one of the following characteristics?

    (A) The morphologic structure of the cell

    (B) The physical form of the antigen that stimulates the eventual response

    (C) The ability of the cell to be clonally selected by antigen; B cells are selected by antigen whereas T cells are not

    (D) The ability to produce a memory response

5. Clonal selection refers to which one of the following?

    (A) Only the ability of B cells to react with specific antigen

    (B) Only the ability of T cells to react with specific antigen

    (C) The nature of the antigen changes, but clonal selection is equally applicable to both T cells and B cells

    (D) The generation of antigen-binding diversity

Note. Abbreviations used in review questions: APCs = antigen presenting cells; IgM = immunoglobulin M; MHC = major histocompatibility complex; TCR = T-cell receptor; IgG = immunoglobulin G.

6. Which one of the following statements best describes the differences between antigen receptors on B and T cells?

   (A) The specificity of the B-cell antigen receptor is randomly generated, while antigen helps instruct the T cell on the construction of the TCR.

   (B) There are no differences in the nature of the antigen that binds to either the B-cell receptor or the TCR because both receptors bind to native, intact antigen.

   (C) The B-cell antigen receptor is capable of directly binding native, un-processed antigen, whereas the TCR requires that the antigen be frag-mented and displayed on a cell-surface MHC molecule.

   (D) The TCR is capable of directly binding native, unprocessed antigen, whereas the B-cell antigen receptor requires that the antigen be fragmented and displayed on a cell-surface MHC molecule.

7. Cytotoxic T lymphocytes recognize foreign antigen in which one of the following conditions?

   (A) The context of class I major MHC molecules

   (B) The context of class II MHC molecules

   (C) The association with the γ-heavy chain of IgG

   (D) The association with the μ-heavy chain of IgM

8. Which one of the following sets of cell-surface molecules is involved in antigen recognition by cytotoxic T cells?

   (A) CD3, CD4, and class II MHC

   (B) CD3, CD4, and class I MHC

   (C) CD3, CD8, and class II MHC

   (D) CD3, CD8, and class I MHC

9. Which one of the following sets of cell-surface molecules is involved in antigen recognition by helper T cells?

   (A) CD3, CD4, and class II MHC

   (B) CD3, CD4, and class I MHC

   (C) CD3, CD8, and class II MHC

   (D) CD3, CD8, and class I MHC

10. Which one of the following is a component of the TCR for antigen?

    (A) CD3

    (B) Lymphocyte membrane-bound IgM

    (C) Class I MHC

    (D) Class II MHC

11. Which one of the following cell-surface structures is found on all nucleated cells and functions in the presentation of intracellular antigen?

    (A) CD4

    (B) CD8

    (C) Class I MHC

    (D) Class II MHC

12. Which one of the following sets of molecules is found on APCs?

(A) Class II MHC and CD8

(B) Class I MHC and CD4

(C) CD8 and CD4

(D) Class I MHC and class II MHC

13. Which one of the following cell-surface molecules is responsible for presenting an extracellular antigen?

(A) CD4

(B) CD3

(C) Class I MHC

(D) Class II MHC

14. Which one of the following cell-surface molecules is responsible for presenting a viral antigen that has infected a cell?

(A) CD4

(B) CD3

(C) Class I MHC

(D) Class II MHC

ANSWERS AND EXPLANATIONS

1. **The answer is B.** APCs require functional lysosomes in which to process antigen. The processing pathway for the class I MHC molecules uses the cytoplasmic proteasomes to process antigen.

2. **The answer is C.** Although B cells can be selected by antigen in the absence of T-cell help, they cannot complete the differentiation process necessary to make antibody without the T cell. The one exception to this is a type of antigen called T-independent antigen. T-independent antigens stimulate IgM responses only.

3. **The answer is C.** In the thymus, the developing T lymphocytes are trained to (1) recognize and bind to self-MHC molecules and (2) control or become tolerant to self-molecules. Therefore, once a T lymphocyte has been selected by antigen, that cell will not respond if either the antigen or the MHC molecule is altered.

4. **The answer is B.** B cells are selected directly by binding antigen. T cells, on the other hand, are selected by antigen that has been processed and presented in the context of the MHC molecule.

5. **The answer is C.** Both B and T lymphocytes respond to specific antigens. The lymphocytes that respond to antigen develop in the absence of antigen and are eventually selected by antigens.

6. **The answer is C.** Both B- and T-cell antigen receptors are structurally similar and are members of the immunoglobulin gene superfamily of molecules. Moreover, antigen-binding specificity of both the TCR and the B-cell receptor are generated by a similar process of gene rearrangement. The major functional difference between these two antigen receptors is in the nature of the antigen that binds to the receptor. B cells bind antigen directly, whereas T lymphocytes bind a processed antigen that is displayed in the context of a cell-surface MHC molecule.

7. **The answer is A.** CD8 cytotoxic T lymphocytes respond to antigen that was synthe-sized inside of the cell and presented on the class I MHC molecule. CD4 helper T lymphocytes respond to antigen that was phagocytized and presented on the class II MHC molecule.

8. **The answer is D.** Cytotoxic T cells display the CD8 differentiation antigen and are selected by the processed antigen that is associated with the class I MHC molecule.

9. **The answer is A.** Helper T cells display the CD4 differentiation antigen and are selected by the processed antigen that is associated with the class II MHC molecule.

10. **The answer is A.** Both the class I and class II MHC molecules are part of the antigen complex. The TCR, however, is associated with CD3 molecules, which aid in the transduction of the signal that is generated when the T cell binds antigen. CD3 molecules are components of the TCR complex and are used as markers to identify T cells.

11. **The answer is C.** CD4 and CD8 are components of the T cell. The class II MHC molecules are found only on selected types of APCs. All nucleated cells, however, express class I MHC molecules.

12. **The answer is D.** APCs are also nucleated cells. Consequently these cell types express both class I and class II MHC molecules.

13. **The answer is D.** Extracellular antigen is processed and presented to CD4 T cells by class II MHC–expressing APCs.

14. **The answer is C.** Intracellular antigen is processed and presented to CD8 T cells by all types of nucleated cells. All nucleated cells express class I MHC molecules.

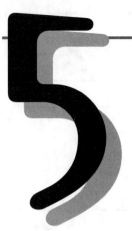

EFFECTOR FUNCTIONS OF THE IMMUNE SYSTEM

INTRODUCTION OF CLINICAL CASE

Mrs. Neilson, a 62-year-old woman, went to see her physician complaining of a very rapid onset of body aches, itchy eyes, coryza, and a slight fever. She had a nonproductive cough, and her lungs were clear to auscultation. A rapid test for influenza was positive for the influenza antigen. In addition, a complete blood cell (CBC) count with differential was performed on a sample of Mrs. Neilson's blood. The results are shown in Table 5-1.

Mrs. Neilson's immune system faced the challenge of responding to an influenza virus infection, much as Jane Cerwinski's system responded to the measles vaccination (see Chap. 4). Mrs. Neilson's infection was complicated by the fact that not only must her immune system identify and remove extracellular virus, but it must also identify cells that are infected with the virus and prevent the continued synthesis of new virus particles. In order to accomplish this, not only must her immune system be able to synthesize antibody capable of removing virus, but it also needs to develop the cytotoxic T lymphocytes (CTLs) that can prevent additional viral replication.

TABLE 5-1 ▶
Mrs. Neilson's White Blood Cell (WBC)
Count with Differential

	Mrs. Neilson	Normal Values
WBC count	$13 \times 10^3/\mu L$	$7-14 \times 10^3/\mu L$
Segmented neutrophils	50%	60%–70%
Banded neutrophils	0%	0%–5%
Lymphocytes	42%	20%–40%
Monocytes	7%	2%–6%
Basophils	0%	0%–1%
Eosinophils	1%	1%–4%

FUNCTIONS OF CD4 T LYMPHOCYTES

This chapter focuses on the functional activities of the lymphocytes and how clonal selection, discussed in Chap. 4, eventually results in the elimination of antigen. Central to all of these responses are the CD4 cells.

To understand the effector functions of the lymphocytes, it is critical, initially, to comprehend the activities of the CD4 helper cells. As depicted in Fig. 5-1, the CD4 T lymphocyte plays a central and regulatory role in the responses of both B lymphocytes and CD8 cytotoxic T lymphocytes. In addition, the CD4 cells can coordinate the responses of a variety of other cell types in response to antigen.

FIGURE 5-1 ▶
Functions of CD4 T Lymphocytes. The CD4 populations of T lymphocytes have a central role in most aspects of immunity. These cells help selected B cells make antibody of the appropriate isotype, provide growth and differentiation signals to the bone marrow that stimulate hematopoiesis, provide growth factors for both CD4 and CD8 lymphocytes, and orchestrate the delayed-type hypersensitivity response.

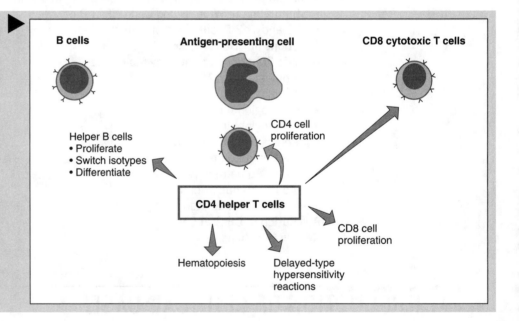

Help for Selected B Cells

When antigen clonally selects a B cell, the B cell is stimulated. This stimulation can be viewed as promoting the resting B lymphocyte from the G_0 phase to the G_1 phase of the cell cycle. However, in order for the selected B cell to respond effectively, it must (1) *proliferate*, create many more daughter cells capable of reacting with the same antigen; (2) *switch isotype*, change from producing immunoglobulin M (IgM) antibody to an antibody isotype better suited for removal of the antigen; and (3) *differentiate*, become either a memory B cell or an antibody-secreting plasma cell (Fig. 5-2). The information necessary to accomplish these cellular changes comes from the CD4 T lymphocyte in the form of *cytokines*. The cytokines represent a diverse group of proteins that express potent paracrine, endocrine, and autocrine activities. If the cytokine is produced by a monocyte,

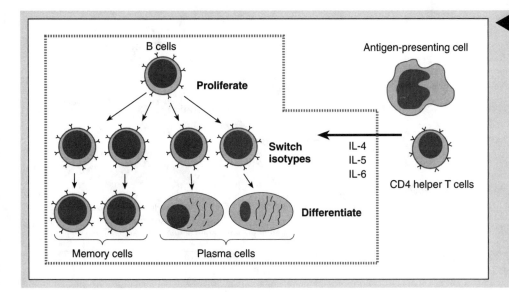

FIGURE 5-2
Role of CD4 T Lymphocytes in Helping B Cells. *Upon selection by antigen, the selected B cell must proliferate, switch antibody isotypes to that which will most effectively eliminate the antigen, and differentiate into either plasma or memory cells. The help for these three events comes from helper T lymphocytes (CD4 cells) in the form of lymphokines. To provide the B-cell growth and differentiation factor activity, the cytokines interleukin-4 (IL-4), -5 (IL-5), and -6 (IL-6) must act in concert. In this case, it is the combination of factors, probably with other as yet unidentified factors, that provides the selected B cells with the appropriate information.*

the term monokine is used, whereas if the cytokine is produced by a lymphocyte, the term lymphokine is applied. However, some cytokines are also given names based on their activities. For example, a monokine that helps direct stem cells to differentiate into granulocytes is called a *granulocyte colony-stimulating factor* (G-CSF). Still another term used in referring to cytokines is *interleukin*. Interleukins can come from different cell types, but the term usually refers to cytokines that provide a signal to, from, or between leukocytes. The task of understanding the nomenclature and function of the cytokines is further complicated because many of these molecules are pluripotent, having both major and minor activities. In addition, some cytokines function both alone and in concert with other cytokines. Moreover, the same cytokine can be produced by many different cells and have multiple target sites of action.

In this chapter, only the major activities of the key cytokines are discussed. The specific cytokines that play a major role in providing help to selected B lymphocytes are interleukin-4 (IL-4), -5 (IL-5), and -6 (IL-6). These cytokines, together with, potentially, other unknown factors, provide the B-cell growth factor and B-cell differentiation factor activities that allow B cells to proliferate, switch isotype, and differentiate.

Cytokines express pluripotent paracrine, endocrine, and autocrine activities.

Help for Selected CD8 Lymphocytes

Like B cells, selected CD8 cytotoxic T cells also need to proliferate to produce both a memory and a substantial cytotoxic T-cell response. Again, this information comes from the CD4 lymphocyte in the form of cytokines. Fig. 5-3 schematically illustrates the kind of help that a CD4 helper T lymphocyte can provide cytotoxic T cells. In this case, the cytokine with T-cell growth factor is interleukin-2 (IL-2).

Help for Selected CD4 Lymphocytes

Not only do CD8 T lymphocytes require IL-2 growth factors from activated CD4 cells to proliferate, but the CD4 cells themselves need to proliferate to produce an effective response that can spread to other locations. In this case, the information needed comes from the clonally selected CD4 cell itself in the form of cytokines. Again, IL-2 provides this information.

Coordinating Delayed-Type Hypersensitivity Reactions

Delayed-type hypersensitivity (DTH) was initially detected as a type of cutaneous reaction that was distinct from the more immediate anaphylactic reactions. These reactions take longer to become visible (24–48 hours) and are characteristically indurated (hard), as opposed to the immediate hypersensitivity reaction, which is edematous. In DTH

FIGURE 5-3 ▶
Role of CD4 Lymphocytes in Helping Cytotoxic T Lymphocytes (CTLs). Upon clonal selection of a CD8 CTL, the selected T cell must proliferate to respond effectively to the antigen. The T-cell growth factor information for proliferation of this selected cell comes in the form of interleukin-2 (IL-2).

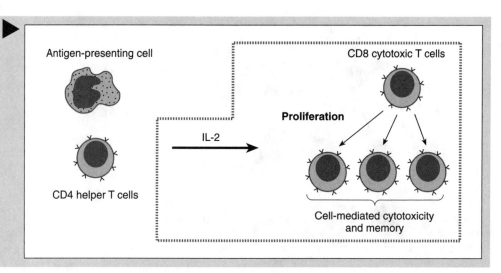

reactions, cytokines elaborated by CD4 T lymphocytes are responsible for recruiting monocytes and lymphocytes to the area of inflammation, activating the monocytes, and preventing them from leaving. In addition, other cells of the innate immune system, such as natural killer (NK) cells and local tissue macrophages, are activated. Nonlymphoid nucleated cells in the area are also stimulated to increase their antigen-processing capability. This entire process can be viewed as a method to recruit a cell-mediated inflammatory response to an area that is localized or isolated from the lymph node. The events in the DTH reaction are schematically illustrated in Fig. 5-4. The CD4 lymphocytes mediating DTH synthesize multiple factors; however, the critical cytokine that is responsible for coordinating DTH reactions is interferon-γ (IFN-γ).

FIGURE 5-4 ▶
Role of CD4 Lymphocytes in Delayed-Type Hypersensitivity (DTH). Interferon-γ (IFN-γ) is the principal cytokine that mediates DTH reactions. When a CD4 helper T lymphocyte (Th1) is clonally selected by a class II MHC–antigen complex, outside of the lymph node or spleen, a DTH reaction usually results. This reaction can be visualized as CD4 cells calling components of the immune system to the site of an antigen challenge. The reaction involves increasing monocyte chemotaxis to the site of the reaction and preventing the infiltrating monocytes from leaving the site. The monocytes are activated to increase their killing capacity, and natural killer (NK) cells in the area are activated to increase their killing capacity. All nucleated cells in the area are stimulated to process and present synthetic products more rapidly, and the density of class I MHC molecules on these cells increases. In addition, the bone marrow stem cell is stimulated to produce more leukocytes. DTH reactions are characterized by the 24–48 hours required to create the indurated swelling, which results from the accumulation of lymphocytes and monocytes. IL = interleukin; TNF = tumor necrosis factor; GM-CSF = granulocyte-monocyte colony-stimulating factor.

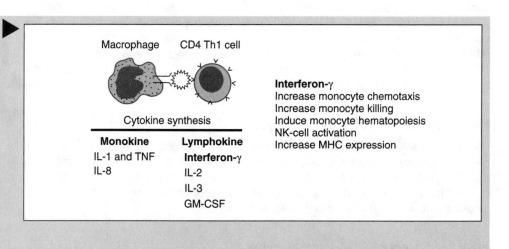

Stimulation of White Blood Cell (WBC) Production

During the course of an inflammatory response, several products are liberated that are toxic to WBCs. These products can be collectively called *lymphotoxins*. In addition, monocytes, polymorphonuclear cells, and other WBC types enter the tissues to fight the infection. This is a one-way trip in which the inflammatory cells die in the tissues. Consequently, it is necessary to signal the bone marrow to replace these lost cells. CD4 T cells, in addition to other cell types, make the growth and differentiation factors for hematopoietic cells. There are several different *colony-stimulating factors* (CSF) such as G-CSF and granulocyte-monocyte–CSF (GM-CSF). The helper T cells also produce interleukin-3 (IL-3), which stimulates the production of all hematopoietic cells.

Th1 and Th2 Populations of Helper T Cells

When all CD4 functions are looked at together, a picture emerges of a cell population that functions by producing critical regulatory cytokines in response to antigen-specific stimulation. The cytokines produced, however, have such diverse activities and activities in different immunological reactions that one cell type cannot make all of the required factors unless there is another control mechanism that directs the CD4 T lymphocyte activity. It is currently thought that there are at least two subpopulations of CD4 T lymphocytes. These populations of helper T cells are called Th1 and Th2 cells. The two cell populations cannot be distinguished from each other based on cell-surface differentiation antigens, and both sets of cells express the T-cell antigen receptor (TCR) and the CD4 differentiation antigen. The cells do differ, however, in the products that are generated. The major Th1 and Th2 products are identified in Table 5-2.

◀ **TABLE 5-2**
Th1 and Th2 Major Cytokines

Cytokines	Th1 Cells	Th2 Cells
IL-3 (hematopoietic growth factor)	+	+
GM-CSF (granulocyte-monocyte colony-stimulating factor)	+	+
IL-2 (T-cell growth factor)	+	−
Interferon-γ (delayed-type hypersensitivity)	+	−
IL-4	−	+
IL-5	−	+
IL-6	−	+
IL-10	−	+

Note. IL = interleukin; Th1, Th2 = helper T-cell populations 1 and 2.

By this point, it should be evident that the Th1 cells are responsible for making the cytokines that mediate DHT reactions, while the Th2 cells are responsible for helping B cells proliferate, differentiate into plasma cells or memory cells, and direct an isotype switch in the B cell to the immunoglobulin E (IgE) isotype. It is not clear, at this writing, if the other antibody isotypes are the result of other, as yet undefined, Th2-like cells or if production of the immunoglobulin G (IgG) and immunoglobulin A (IgA) isotypes is the result of mixtures of Th1 and Th2 cells.

FUNCTIONS OF CD8 EFFECTOR CELLS

The CD8 cells are cytotoxic. The cell recognizes processed antigen in the context of the class I major histocompatibility complex (MHC) molecule. When the processed antigen–class I MHC initially selects the appropriate CD8 cell, the CD8 cell is activated, can receive help in the form of T-cell growth factors, and can then proliferate. In this case, the growth factor is IL-2 and the Th1 CD4 cell is the primary source.

When normal tissue expressing different class I MHC molecules is transplanted from one individual to another, there is a rapid rejection of the tissue, although all proteins except the MHC molecules may be identical. Why is there a more rapid tissue rejection than when the nonidentity is in some other protein?

Upon binding to a target cell, the CD8 CTL secretes molecules called porins, or perforins, that function very much like the lytic component of the complement system. Therefore, interaction of a CTL with a somatic cell expressing antigen on the class I MHC molecule results in both antigen-specific and class I MHC–specific lysis of the target cell. It must be emphasized that, if either the antigen is changed or the class I MHC molecule is altered, the CD8 cell will not lyse the target displaying the antigen.

In addition to lysis of the target cell, nucleases are activated by the interaction of the CD8 cell and the antigen-expressing target cell. The nucleases destroy the nucleic acids that contained coding information for the target antigen. Not only is the cell destroyed, but the molecular memory of the antigen (nucleic acid) is also destroyed. Fig. 5-5 schematically illustrates the events in the killing of Mrs. Neilson's influenza-infected cells by CTLs.

FIGURE 5-5 ▶
Activity of CD8 Cytotoxic T Lymphocytes (CTLs). CTLs are selected by the class I MHC–antigen complex. Upon selection, the CTL begins producing and secreting perforins. These molecules, which resemble the membrane attack complex of the complement system, lyse the target antigen–MHC-expressing cell. In addition to cell lysis, the interaction between the target cell and the CD8 CTL activates nucleases, which digest the nuclear material in the target cell.

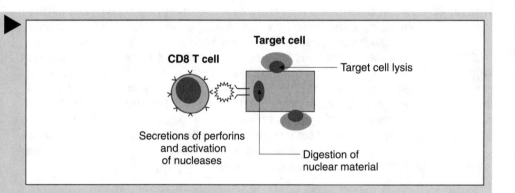

GENERIC FUNCTIONS OF ANTIBODY MOLECULES

For an optimal response to her influenza infection and to prevent future infections with the identical virus more efficiently, killing the virally infected cells is not sufficient. Mrs. Neilson also needs mechanisms in place that can remove virus particles from the extracellular fluids before they can infect another cell. CTLs cannot perform this task because they do not physically bind to the intact nonprocessed viral particle. In this case, antibody is necessary to tag extracellular viral particles for removal by the phagocytic cells of the reticuloendothelial system.

The antibody molecule (Fig. 5-6) needs to be considered a bifunctional molecule. The most obvious function is to bind antigen. The sites of antigen binding are located in the antigen-binding fragment (Fab) portions of the molecule. However, binding to a target structure is not always sufficient to eliminate or neutralize the structure. If the target is bacteria, simply putting an additional molecule on the bacterial surface may do absolutely nothing to the bacteria in terms of killing them or preventing their adherence or reproduction. To kill a microorganism or promote its disposal, the antibody molecule must recruit other biologic mechanisms.

A second function of the antibody molecule is, then, to interact with a set of generic mechanisms to kill, remove, or detoxify the target antigen. These other biologic functions of the antibody include precipitation or agglutination, activation of complement, and opsonization of particles for phagocytic cells. In addition, some antibodies function by inactivating bacterial toxins, thus preventing adherence or absorption of microorganisms. Each of the antibody isotypes has its own set of biologic functions, and, depending on the nature of the antigen and route of exposure, the CD4 T cell helps the B lymphocyte switch to the proper antibody isotype.

Immunoglobulin M

The IgM molecule plays two entirely different roles in the immune response. One role is the antigen receptor on B lymphocytes, which has been discussed. A second role for the

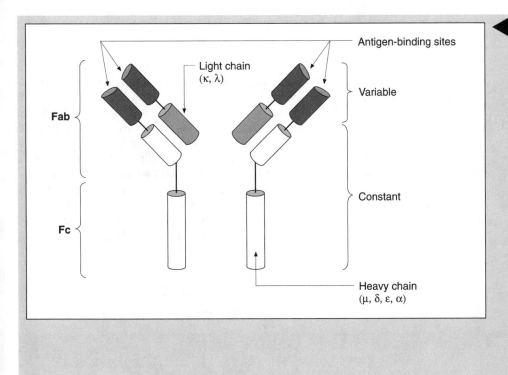

FIGURE 5-6
Generic Antibody Molecule. *The antibody is a bifunctional molecule. One function of the molecule is to bind antigen. This function is located in the variable section of the antibody. The term variable is derived from comparing amino acid sequences of antibodies to different antigens. A second function of the molecule is to activate methods to remove antigen or carry out the antibodies' other biologic functions. These functions include: activating complement, binding to and directing phagocytes to an antibody-coated cell, precipitating and agglutinating antigen, and transporting or inhibiting transport across membranes. The molecule is composed of four polypeptide chains, two identical heavy chains and two identical light chains. The different isotypes of antibody have different heavy chains. IgM contains a heavy chain called a μ-chain. The IgG heavy chain is a γ-chain. The IgE heavy chain is an ε-chain, while the IgA heavy chain is an α-chain. The light chain for all different classes of antibody can be either a κ-chain or a λ-chain. The different antibody isotypes have different physical and biologic properties and function differently in the removal of antigen. Fab = antigen-binding fragment; Fc = fragment without antigen-binding site.*

IgM molecule is in the primary response to antigen. Fig. 5-7 illustrates the structure of the secreted form of the IgM molecule. To provide a first response, the IgM molecule must be synthesized rapidly. It must readily bind to foreign structures even when there is not a perfect match between antigen and antibody. The pentameric design of the molecule, with 10 antigen-binding sites, helps offset an imperfect match with antigen by aggregating multiple binding sites into one molecule. This also makes the IgM molecule exceedingly efficient in activating the complement system. In addition to forming immune complexes with low-affinity antibody and efficient complement activation, the polymeric structure of the molecule allows a single IgM molecule to aggregate, or agglutinate, several antigens into a significantly larger structure that can resemble a particle. Because phagocytic cells, including antigen-presenting cells (APCs), are very efficient in phagocytizing particles, the IgM immune complexes are readily taken up for antigen processing and presentation.

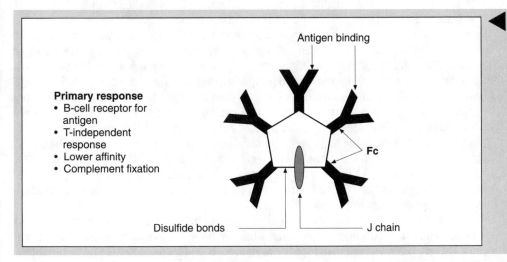

FIGURE 5-7
Immunoglobulin M. *The IgM molecule has two major functions. One function is the B-cell receptor for antigen. On the B-cell surface the molecule is a monomer. However, the secreted form of the molecule is a polymer in which five monomeric IgM molecules are covalently joined with an additional polypeptide chain, called a joining (J) chain. The secreted IgM molecule is the major component of a primary antibody response and is efficient in activating the complement system. Fab = antigen-binding fragment; Fc = fragment without antigen-binding site.*

Immunoglobulin G

The immunoglobulin molecule that looks most like the generic antibody molecule is IgG (Fig. 5-8). Unlike IgM, IgG and the remaining immunoglobulin molecules are products of a secondary immune response. This means that T-cell help and immunologic memory have been generated. Although IgG can fix complement and can agglutinate and precipitate, as do the IgM molecules, it is not as efficient. IgG, however, works very elegantly with the phagocytes of the innate immune system. Several cell types, including monocytes, macrophages, polymorphonuclear neutrophils (PMNs), and the NK cells, possess a cell-surface receptor for the Fc fragment of the IgG immunoglobulin (FcR) that aids in the phagocytic and killing function. The IgG molecule is the product of a secondary immune response. This means that, following initial clonal selection, there has been cell growth and potential repeated clonal selection, allowing the antibody affinity to increase. Consequently, IgG and all other antibodies of the secondary immune response can, potentially, bind antigen with greater affinities than can the IgM molecules observed in the initial response.

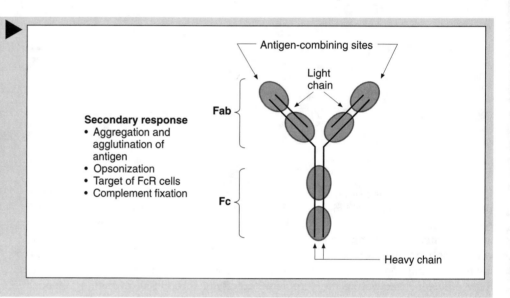

Figure 5-8

Immunoglobulin G. *The IgG molecule looks like the generic antibody molecule in Fig. 5-6. The molecule is found primarily in the serum and lymph as a result of secondary immune responses, and it has a relatively long half-life of approximately 3 weeks. The IgG molecule functions in the precipitation and agglutination of antigen. It efficiently opsonizes particles for phagocytosis, and although not as efficient as IgM, the IgG molecule also fixes complement. In addition, in humans and some other species, the IgG molecule is passively transferred across the placenta to provide passive immunologic protection of the newborn. Fab = antigen-binding fragment; Fc = fragment without antigen-binding site; FcR = cell-surface receptor for Fc component.*

Immunoglobulin E

Like IgG, IgE is a product of the secondary immune response. A schematic illustration of the antibody is represented in Fig. 5-9. IgE is the antibody molecule that is responsible for allergic and anaphylactic reactions. It is referred to by several other names, including reagenic antibody, reagin, and cytophilic antibody. This last term provides a very useful indication of how this particular antibody functions. IgE antibodies bind avidly to mast cells and basophils through the Fc portion of the antibody and an Fc$_\varepsilon$ receptor on the mast cell or basophil. In the presence of antigen, two IgE antibodies with specificity for that antigen are cross-linked, and the resulting cross-link triggers the mast cell or basophil to release its preformed granules, containing histamine and other vasoactive amines (degranulation). In addition to promoting degranulation, the cross-linking of IgE antibodies on mast cells or basophils initiates the synthesis and release of inflammatory lipid mediators, proteases, and inflammatory cytokines. Together, these substances are referred to as the slow-reacting substance of anaphylaxis, and they function to further enhance and maintain the localized inflammation. Although the serum concentration of IgE antibody is extremely low and the molecule has a relatively short circulating half-life, it must be remembered that serum IgE antibody is not the major pool of the molecule. The bulk of IgE antibody is cell bound, and as a cell-bound antibody it appears to have a much longer duration in the body.

The function of IgE antibody can be likened to that of a sentry. In the presence of antigen and mast cell- or basophil-bound IgE antibody, the resulting degranulation promotes a very dramatic call to recruit the remainder of the immune system (inflammation).

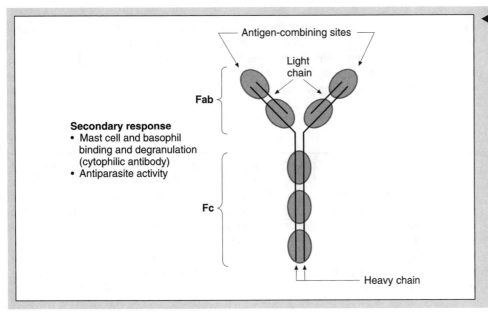

Secondary response
- Mast cell and basophil binding and degranulation (cytophilic antibody)
- Antiparasite activity

FIGURE 5-9
Immunoglobulin E. The IgE molecule looks like the generic antibody molecule but has a slightly longer Fc region. The molecule binds avidly to an Fc_ε receptor, found on both mast cells and basophils. The circulating concentration of the molecule is extremely low; however, the synthetic rate and the concentration of cell-bound IgE antibody is substantial. The molecule functions in anaphylactic reactions. When two IgE molecules bound to mast cells are cross-linked by antigen, the mast cell is triggered to degranulate, releasing histamine and other preformed mediators.

Immunoglobulin A

The third antibody involved in the secondary immune response is IgA. This antibody is associated with mucosal immunity. Although IgA is one of the minor serum antibodies in terms of concentration, it is the major antibody in terms of the total amount synthesized per day. It has been estimated that approximately 70% of our daily antibody synthesis is devoted to IgA. The structure of the mucosal form of IgA is illustrated in Fig. 5-10. This antibody contains two additional polypeptide chains. The joining (J) chain is identical to that found in IgM, the other polymeric antibody molecule. The secretory piece, on the other hand, is unique to the mucosal form of the IgA molecule. This additional polypeptide chain provides the IgA molecule with its extreme chemical stability and allows it to function in the harsh mucosal environment. Monomeric and dimeric forms of IgA (without the attached secretory piece) are also detected in the blood. These antibody isotypes have several biologically critical roles. They do not appear to mediate antibody-dependent cell-mediated cytotoxicity reactions, and although they can potentially agglutinate or aggregate an antigen, there is little evidence that it is a major mechanism by which the antibodies function. The IgA antibody appears to function in two different modes. One mode limits adherence and colonization by both bacteria and virus. The IgA molecule can block the actions of some bacterial toxins and effectively prevent adsorp-

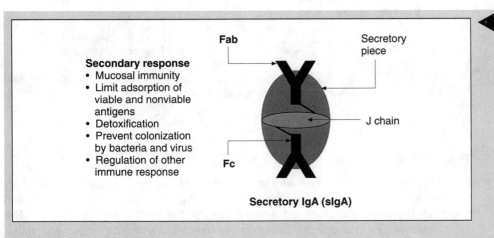

Secondary response
- Mucosal immunity
- Limit adsorption of viable and nonviable antigens
- Detoxification
- Prevent colonization by bacteria and virus
- Regulation of other immune response

Secretory IgA (sIgA)

FIGURE 5-10
Immunoglobulin A. The IgA molecule takes on multiple forms. It is found as a monomeric molecule and as a dimeric molecule, in which the two monomers are joined together by an additional polypeptide joining (J) chain. This is the same J chain found in IgM, the other polymeric antibody. In addition, dimeric IgA is associated with a fourth glycopeptide called the secretory piece. IgA is the antibody responsible for mucosal immunity. IgA limits adsorption of both viable and nonviable antigen, it detoxifies bacterial toxins, it prevents colonization by bacteria and virus, and it performs unidentified regulatory functions in other immune reactions.

tion of microorganisms and macromolecular (antigenic) components in foods and other environmental antigens. The second major function of IgA appears to be in the regulation of IgG and cell-mediated immune responses to environmental and food antigens. Generally, an active IgA response to an antigen implies that there is a low IgG or cell-mediated response to the same antigen. Similarly, a high IgG or cell-mediated response to an antigen implies a low IgA response.

HYPERSENSITIVITY REACTIONS

The immune system's response to either humoral or cellular antigen is vigorous and capable of activating complement and recruiting phagocytic and granulocytic cells. However, these reactions can occur at the expense of healthy tissue. Consequently, it is not unexpected that, during an immune response, there is damage to healthy tissue. This tissue damage is called a *hypersensitivity reaction*. Based upon the immunologic mechanisms involved in the response, these reactions are separated into four distinct categories.

Type I: Immediate

Type I hypersensitivity reactions include tissue damage resulting from immediate anaphylactic reactions. These reactions can be initiated either by the IgE system or by components of the complement cascade (Fig. 5-11). Tissue damage results from the rapid edematous swelling caused by the vasoactive amines. In addition, the infiltration of inflammatory cells, caused by the slow-reacting substances, compounds the tissue damage. Moreover, the major basic protein found in the eosinophil granules appears to have a toxic effect on many different cell types.

FIGURE 5-11 ▶

Type I Hypersensitivity Reaction (Immediate). Tissue damage caused by IgE reactions are classified as anaphylactic or type I hypersensitivity reactions. In these reactions, IgE antibody bound to Fc receptors (FcRε) on either mast cells or basophils, when cross-linked by antigen, triggers the cell to release its preformed granules containing histamine and initiates the synthesis of lipid mediators (prostaglandins and leukotrienes), inflammatory cytokines, and eosinophil chemotactic factors. Together, these factors trigger tissue edema and leukocyte infiltration, all of which cause tissue damage. In addition, the major basic protein found in eosinophil granules has potent toxic activity. This response can be viewed as an emergency signal that recruits the immune system and initiates an inflammatory response at the site of an antigen interaction with IgE.

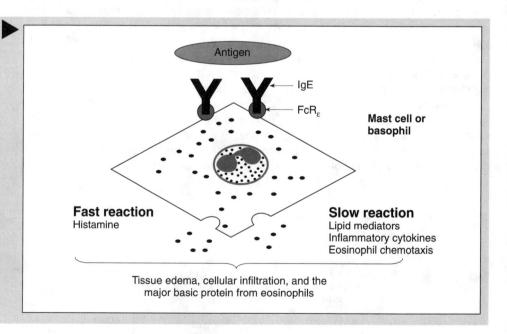

Type II: Autoantibody

Type II hypersensitivity reactions refer to the damage caused by antibody or autoantibody to a normal, healthy cell. In this case autoantibody, usually IgM or IgG, coats and opsonizes the target structure, providing a site for the fixation of complement. The opsonized surface will expose the Fc portions of the antibody molecule, allowing phagocytic cells to engulf and kill the target structure. If the structure is too large to be phagocytosed, products of the activated phagocytes are liberated into the environment, resulting in further damage to adjacent tissue. The fixation of complement adds to the tissue damage by initiating anaphylactic responses, opsonizing the target structure with the C3b component of complement, and even lysing the target structure by the formation of the membrane attack complex. The mechanisms leading to tissue damage in the type II hypersensitivity reactions are illustrated in Fig. 5-12.

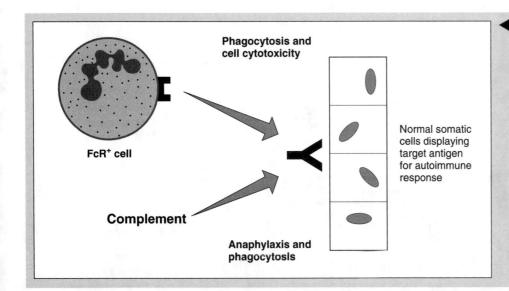

FIGURE 5-12
Type II Hypersensitivity Reaction (Autoantibody). *When an antibody is directed to a target tissue, the tissue-fixed antigen– antibody complex can activate complement, and it or its resulting inflammatory activities opsonize the target tissue for phagocytosis by Fc-receptor-positive (FcR$^+$) phagocytes. In both cases, the tissue that has been decorated with the antibody is destroyed.*

Type III: Immune Complex

Type III hypersensitivity reactions involve mechanisms identical to those described for the type II hypersensitivity reactions; however, the nature of the antigen is different. Whereas, in type II reactions, the immune complex that stimulates the response is an autoantibody bound to a target cell, in type III reactions, the target is an immune complex from a response at a distant location that is trapped in a tissue. Different antigen– antibody complexes have different affinities for tissues such as skin, joints, and kidney glomerulus, and they can lodge in these structures. This results in an immune-complex type of disease, illustrated in Fig. 5-13.

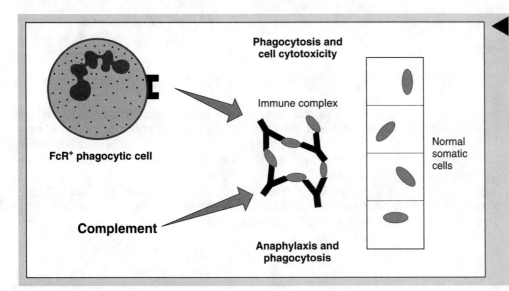

FIGURE 5-13
Type III Hypersensitivity Reaction (Immune Complex). *When antigen–antibody complexes are formed as the result of a successful immunologic reaction, they sometimes are of appropriate size or have chemical characteristics that prevent them from being cleared efficiently by the reticuloendothelial system. In such cases, the complexes lodge in capillary beds. The aggregated immune complexes activate both complement and Fc-receptor-positive (FcR+) killer cells in order to clear the complex. The result of this activation involves not only clearing the complex but also tissue damage.*

Type IV: Cell-mediated

Cell-mediated reactions resulting in tissue damage are collectively referred to as type IV hypersensitivity reactions. These reactions can involve either CD4 Th1 cells (hypersensitivity DTH) [Fig. 5-14], or CD8 CTLs (Fig. 5-15). Tissue damage resulting from activated CD8 cell function is relatively easy to understand because the target cell expressing the antigen is destroyed. Even cells infected with a slow-growing, or nonlytic, virus are rapidly destroyed by CTLs, and in some infections the CD8 cytotoxic response to a virus causes far more tissue damage than the virus does.

FIGURE 5-14 ▶

Type IV Hypersensitivity Reaction (Delayed-Type Hypersensitivity [DTH]). There are two forms of type IV hypersensitivity reactions, and both are considered to be cell-mediated immunity. One form of the type IV reaction is DTH. In this reaction, interferon-γ from the CD4 Th1 cell increases monocyte chemotaxis to the site of antigen presentation, as well as increasing monocyte-killing functions, activating natural killer (NK) cells and increasing the expression of MHC molecules. After 24–48 hours, there is a generalized increase in macrophages and lymphocytes in the area, and normal tissues are damaged by the activated cells and granule contents that are released. With chronic exposure to antigen and chronic stimulation of DTH reactions, the monocytes isolate the antigen source, resulting in the formation of a structure called a granuloma.

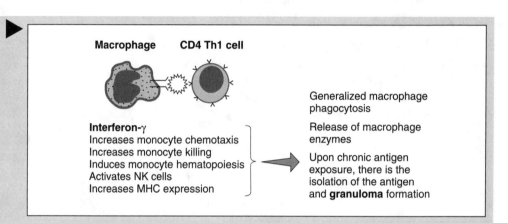

FIGURE 5-15 ▶

Type IV Hypersensitivity Reaction (Cytotoxic T Lymphocytes [CTLs]). The second form of a type IV hypersensitivity reaction is due to CTLs. In this reaction, CTLs detect antigen expressed by either normal or infected host cells, and they kill the host cells. If a sufficient number of host cells are destroyed, the structural integrity or the biologic function conferred by the cells is compromised.

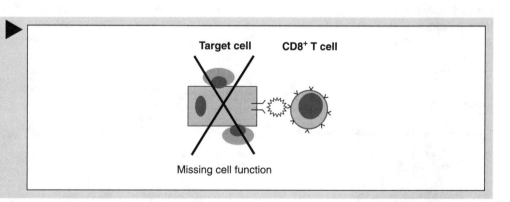

Damage caused by DTH reactions can be more difficult to understand and can take on many different forms. DTH reactions, through the activities of IFN-γ, activate all cells in a local area and can subvert their normal functions. In addition, DTH reactions recruit and activate monocytes, which results in killing or removing not only the offending antigen but also normal tissue.

In the case of a chronic DTH reaction, where the antigen source is either large or sequestered from the immune system, the DTH response isolates the antigen. This results in the formation of a structure called a *granuloma*.

RESOLUTION OF CLINICAL CASE

Mrs. Neilson's condition exemplifies many of the above reactions. Initially the influenza virus infected the epithelial lining of her bronchial mucosal tissues. The virus was able to reproduce in her cells and spread beyond the initial site of infection. CTLs were selected by the class I MHC–antigen complex in her tissues. These CD8 cells, after receiving help in the form of IL-2, were able to proliferate, seed all of Mrs. Neilson's tissues, and kill virally infected cells. Extracellular virus was also taken up by the tissue histiocytes and presented to CD4 Th1 cells. In addition, some of the virus or virus fragments from lysed infected tissue were directed to the local nodes, where both B lymphocytes and Th lymphocytes were clonally selected. This resulted in antibody production. The antibody, initially IgM and eventually IgG, was then able to mark extracellular antigens for removal by tissue phagocytes and prevent the virus from infecting more cells.

The influenza virus infects the mature differentiated epithelial cells of the bronchial tree. These cells constitute an important component of the innate immune system because they develop the cilia that help prevent access of pathogens to the lungs. Not only did Mrs. Neilson's immune response to influenza-infected cells prevent continued viral replication, but the tissue damage associated with the response killed the cells, which provided a critical anatomic barrier that prevented microorganisms from gaining access to her lungs.

The effector functions of the immune response to antigen are summarized in Fig. 5-16. These responses involve a coordinated effort of multiple tissue types, both immune and nonimmune. The immune system orchestrates this response and utilizes all the toxic mechanisms of both innate and acquired immunity to prevent continued viral replication and to remove virus. How this coordination is accomplished is the focus of Chap. 6.

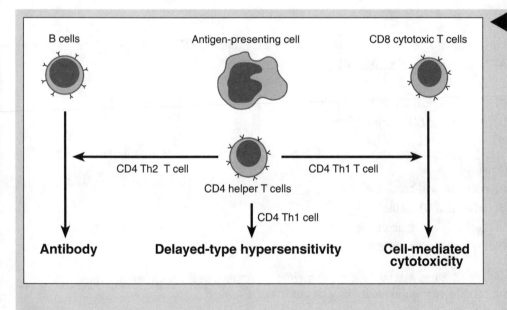

◀ *FIGURE 5-16*

Summary of Lymphocyte Functions. A cell central to all immune responses is the CD4 helper T cell. The Th2-type of helper T cells helps B cells efficiently make antibody, secondary responses, and memory responses. The Th1-type of helper T cells both mediates delayed-type hypersensitivity reactions and helps cytotoxic T cells (CTLs) proliferate, resulting in a memory-CTL response. Removal of the helper T-cell population significantly compromises the entire immune response. Given the major roles that products generated by the formation of a complex between the antigen-presenting cell (APC), antigen fragment, and CD4 cell (trimolecular complex) have in the eventual immune response, it is not unexpected that this is the target of a significant amount of research directed at understanding and controlling the immune response.

REVIEW QUESTIONS

Directions: For each of the following questions, choose the **one best** answer.

1. Which of the following is a function of the CD4 population of T lymphocytes?
   (A) Synthesizing IgM
   (B) Helping B lymphocytes change antibody isotypes
   (C) Helping antigen clonally select B lymphocytes
   (D) Helping antigen clonally select T lymphocytes

2. Which of the following tests would allow an investigator to distinguish between Th1 and Th2 cells?
   (A) Determine the cell-surface density of the CD3 differentiation antigen
   (B) Assess the cell-surface expression of the CD4 differentiation antigen
   (C) Assess the cell-surface expression of the CD8 differentiation antigen
   (D) Identify the cytokine products of the activated cells

3. When a B lymphocyte has been selected by a T-dependent antigen, which one of the following activities is dependent on help from T lymphocytes?
   (A) Proliferation of the B lymphocyte
   (B) Generating the diversity of the B-cell antigen receptor
   (C) Expression of cell-surface IgM
   (D) Expression of B-cell class II MHC molecules

4. Which of the following sets of cells are the most abundant in a DTH response?
   (A) Neutrophils and eosinophils
   (B) Lymphocytes and monocytes
   (C) CD8 lymphocytes and neutrophils
   (D) B cells and CD4 T cells

5. Cytotoxic T lymphocytes effect lysis of target cells using which one of the following mechanisms?
   (A) Antibody and complement
   (B) IFN-γ and NK cells
   (C) Antibody and macrophage
   (D) Perforins and nucleases

6. In a patient who has a total lack of functional T lymphocytes, which one of the following conditions would most likely be observed?
   (A) All immune functions would be missing.
   (B) All T-cell responses would be missing; however, the humoral response would be normal.
   (C) Only antibody of the IgM isotype would be present in the serum.
   (D) Only antibody of the IgG isotype would be present in the serum.

Note. Abbreviations used in the review questions: IgM = immunoglobulin M; MHC = major histocompatibility complex; DTH = delayed-type hypersensitivity; IFN-γ = interferon-γ; NK = natural killer; IgG = immunoglobulin G; IgE = immunoglobulin E; IgA = immunoglobulin A; RBCs = red blood cells; CTLs = cytotoxic T lymphocytes.

7. A patient who sustained a severe snake bite was brought to the emergency room. He was given equine antivenom gamma globulin and responded well to the treatment. Within 5 days the patient developed a slight fever and hives. Examination of the skin lesion revealed the presence of an edematous infiltrate with polymorphonuclear neutrophils. Which one of the following responses is most consistent with these data?

   (A) The patient has a primary humoral immune response to the gamma globulin.

   (B) The patient has a secondary humoral immune response to the gamma globulin.

   (C) The patient is experiencing a direct toxic effect of the equine gamma globulin.

   (D) The patient has a secondary cell-mediated immune response to the gamma globulin.

8. A 56-year-old woman presented with a normochromic-normocytic anemia. Serum levels of bilirubin (direct) were elevated, and the level of serum complement component C3 was significantly reduced. There were normal levels of complement component factor B. Which one of the following conditions is most consistent with these data?

   (A) The patient has an inability to produce complement component C3.

   (B) The patient has a humoral immune response against her own RBCs.

   (C) The patient has a cytotoxic T-cell response against her own RBCs.

   (D) The patient has a DTH response against her own RBCs.

9. A 5-year-old boy has been seen repeatedly by his physician for bacterial infections (*Staphylococcus*, *E. coli*, *Pseudomonas*, pneumococcus), which have been successfully controlled only with the aid of antibiotics. These infections have consistently produced multiple and disseminated granulomas. The patient has high levels of serum antibody specific for these organisms, and there are the normal numbers of cells reported in the complete blood count. During the bacterial infections, the segmented neutrophil population increases. Which one of the following conditions is most consistent with this patient's clinical presentation?

   (A) The patient has an error in the ability to produce antibody.

   (B) There is a problem in the patient's CD4 cell function.

   (C) There is a problem in the patient's CD8 cell function.

   (D) The patient's neutrophils cannot efficiently kill the bacteria.

   (E) The patient cannot mount a DTH response.

10. Which one of the following types of hypersensitivity reaction best describes hemolytic disease of the newborn caused by blood group incompatibility?

   (A) Immediate

   (B) Autoantibody

   (C) Immune complex

   (D) Cell-mediated

11. Which of the following characterizes the principal difference between cytotoxic antibody (type II hypersensitivity) and immune complex hypersensitivity (type III hypersensitivity)?

   (A) Isotype of the antibody

   (B) Distribution of antigen–antibody complexes

   (C) Participation of complement

   (D) Participation of T cells

12. Which group of cells is most likely to be lysed when treated with anti-CD4 antibody and complement?

   (A) CTLs

   (B) Macrophages

   (C) Helper T cells

   (D) B cells

   (E) Neutrophils

13. CTLs are best characterized by which of the following cell-surface markers?

   (A) CD4

   (B) CD3

   (C) CD8

   (D) Surface IgM

14. A patient suffering from a bacterial infection received a penicillin injection and almost immediately experienced respiratory distress and fell into unconsciousness. This reaction is most likely mediated by which of the following immune effector mechanisms?

   (A) CTLs

   (B) IgG

   (C) IgE

   (D) IgA

   (E) DTH T cells

15. Which of the following biologic activities is associated with the Fc fragment of an IgG molecule?

   (A) Complement C3 convertase activity

   (B) Binding to phagocytes

   (C) Antigen binding

   (D) Stimulation of mast cells

16. On the first day of medical school, a sample of purified protein derivative from *Mycobacterium tuberculosis* was injected into a student's skin. If the student had been previously exposed to tuberculosis, which of the following responses would be observed at the injection site?

   (A) Immediate (less than 2 minutes) erythema and edematous swelling lasting 24–48 hours

   (B) Deposition of immune complexes and the fixation of complement over the next 24–48 hours

   (C) Indurated swelling and erythema developing over the next 24–48 hours, resulting primarily from the accumulation of neutrophils

   (D) Indurated swelling and erythema developing over the next 24–48 hours, resulting primarily from the accumulation of monocytes and lymphocytes

   (E) Activation and accumulation of CD8 cytotoxic T lymphocytes at the injection site over the next 24–48 hours

17. A positive DTH tuberculin skin test reaction indicates which of the following conditions?

   (A) A humoral immune response has occurred.

   (B) A cell-mediated immune response has occurred.

   (C) Both the T- and B-cell systems are functional.

   (D) Only the B-cell system is functional.

18. A patient became ill 10 days ago with a viral disease. Laboratory examination revealed that the patient's antibodies against this virus have a high ratio of IgM to IgG. What is the correct conclusion?

   (A) It is unlikely that the patient has encountered this organism previously.

   (B) The patient is predisposed to atopic allergies.

   (C) The information given is irrelevant to previous antigen exposure.

   (D) It is likely that the patient has an autoimmune disease.

ANSWERS AND EXPLANATIONS

1. The answer is B. Whereas CD4 cells have multiple roles in the development of the humoral response, antigen alone will select the appropriate B lymphocyte, and the antigen–MHC complex will select the appropriate T lymphocyte. Once selected, however, T-cell help is necessary for proliferation, isotype switching, and differentiation.

2. The answer is D. Th1 and Th2 cells exhibit identical cell-surface markers. It is, therefore, difficult to impossible to distinguish between them until the cell is stimulated and begins making the cytokines that are unique to each cell type.

3. The answer is A. After clonal selection, all of the necessary steps to produce a humoral response require T-cell help. The one exception to this statement is the unique type of antigen called a T-independent antigen. In the case of a T-independent antigen there is no memory or isotype switching. The other distractors in this question relate to antigen-independent events in B-cell ontogeny.

4. The answer is B. DTH reactions result in the accumulation of primarily lymphocytes and monocytes.

5. The answer is D. Antibody works with either complement or Fc-receptor-positive phagocytes to lyse target cells. IFN-γ mediates DTH reactions, while the CTLs lyse target cells using perforins, a type of molecule that resembles the membrane-attack complex of the complement system. In addition, nuclear material is destroyed by the activation of nucleases.

6. The answer is C. The clonal selection of B cells does not depend on T-cell help, however, subsequent development of the selected B cell requires the T lymphocyte. In the scenario outlined in the question, one would not expect to find a memory response or isotype switching to IgG, IgE, or IgA. However, B cells are still capable of responding to T-independent antigens. Consequently, only IgM is found in the serum.

7. The answer is B. To answer this question, an understanding of timing is critical. A primary immune response generally takes 12–18 days to develop. Five days is too rapid a response to be considered a primary response. The second major factor to consider is that this response causes the accumulation of neutrophils at multiple sites, implicating a humoral response as opposed to cellular responses.

8. The answer is B. The elevated bilirubin indicates a pathology, possibly involving lysis of RBCs. The decreased C3 level indicates activation of the complement system; however, this datum alone does not indicate which of the two complement pathways have been activated. The normal levels of serum complement factor B indicate that the alternate pathway is not activated; therefore, one would expect the antibody-dependent classic pathway to be activated.

9. **The answer is D.** The patient is suffering from repeated bacterial infections, which are normally controlled by antibody immunity. In this case, the patient has elevated levels of specific antibody, indicating that he can make an appropriate antibody response. Therefore, there must be a problem either with the ability of the neutrophils to respond appropriately or, if they can respond, with their killing functions. This second possibility is consistent with the data in this case. The choices referring to select problems in cell-mediated immunity are inconsistent with the data. The patient's CD4 cells are working and responding to the organisms as evidenced by the numerous granulomas. CTLs would not be expected to respond to extracellular organisms.

10. **The answer is B.** In hemolytic disease of the newborn, maternal IgG antibody (secondary response) to fetal blood group antigens crosses the placenta and can coat newborn RBCs. These opsonized RBCs are destroyed, primarily by phagocytosis.

11. **The answer is B.** Identical mechanisms of complement activation and phagocytosis are used to remove antigen in both cases. However, in type II reactions, the antibody is directed to a cell-surface target antigen, while in type III reactions, immune complexes that lodge in capillaries activate the response.

12. **The answer is C.** In the list of cells included in this question, only helper T lymphocytes express the CD4 molecule. Cell-surface antigen–antibody complexes can then activate complement via the classic pathway to effect cell lysis.

13. **The answer is C.** Only the CTLs express the CD8 molecule.

14. **The answer is C.** Immediate hypersensitivity reactions are the result of IgE molecules. This is a secondary immune response, in which mast cell- (or basophil-) bound IgE antibody is cross-linked by antigen, causing the immediate degranulation of the mast cell. The symptoms in the question are the direct result of histamine, one of the contents of mast cell granules.

15. **The answer is B.** The antibody's antigen-binding site is contained within the variable portion of the molecule, which resides in the amino terminal portion. Although the Fc portion of the antibody can initiate the formation of C3 convertase, it is not associated with the enzyme. Stimulation of mast cells requires the participation of the IgE antibody.

16. **The answer is D.** This is the classic definition of a DTH reaction. The antigen is administered in the skin, and only the local reaction is evaluated. The indurated nature of the reaction indicates that lymphocytes and monocytes were drawn to the site of antigen application. If neutrophils were brought to the area, that would produce a more edematous reaction and implicate antigen–antibody complexes.

17. **The answer is B.** DTH is an excellent method to evaluate the functioning of the CD4 population of cells. This reaction provides little help in evaluating the functioning of the B-cell component of immunity.

18. **The answer is A.** The high IgM-to-IgG ratio implies that the sample was taken early in the response to an antigen, before a significant secondary response could develop.

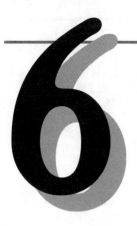

COORDINATION OF THE IMMUNE RESPONSE: MAJOR CYTOKINES

CHAPTER OUTLINE

INTRODUCTION OF CLINICAL CASE

Over the past 4 days, Mrs. Neilson, the patient in Chap. 5, continued to improve. However, on the fifth day she started feeling worse. She developed a high fever and cough. Moreover, she produced significant amounts of sputum containing pneumococcal bacteria and neutrophils. By the sixth day, she was short of breath, and she was rushed to her physician when she noticed blood in her sputum.

Physical examination revealed a woman in respiratory distress. She was febrile, cyanotic, and lethargic. An evaluation of her blood showed lower than normal oxygen saturation. The results of a white blood cell (WBC) count taken at the

> **Erythrocyte Sedimentation Rate**
> During an inflammatory process, altered chemical properties of the inflammatory serum allow erythrocytes to aggregate and, as a result, sediment more rapidly.

time of her evaluation are shown in Table 6-1. An additional test, the erythrocyte sedimentation rate (ESR), was ordered by her physician. This test demonstrated a significantly faster sedimentation of erythrocytes than observed in healthy individuals.

CYTOKINES

Mrs. Neilson's immune response to the pneumococcus requires a coordinated response from several organ systems. The immune system signals the thermoregula-

> What major factor put Mrs. Neilson at increased risk for acquiring a pneumococcal infection?

tory center of the brain to increase the body temperature dramatically and alter the

TABLE 6-1 ▶
Mrs. Neilson's White Blood Cell (WBC) Count.

	Mrs. Neilson	Normal Values
WBC count	$19 \times 10^3/\mu L$	$7-14 \times 10^3/\mu L$
Segmented neutrophils	75%	60%–70%
Banded neutrophils	1%	0%–5%
Lymphocytes	19%	20%–40%
Monocytes	4%	2%–6%
Basophils	0%	0%–1%
Eosinophils	1%	1%–4%

autonomic nervous responses associated with fever. The immune response stimulates the liver to alter the amount and type of proteins synthesized and rapidly changes the WBC count, bringing neutrophils into the area of the pneumococcal infection. In addition, and not as evident in the patient presentation, there are changes in the structure of the endothelial cells in the area of the inflammation. The activity of the bone marrow has been altered to increase the synthesis of granulocytes, monocytes, and lymphocytes. The hypothalamus has been stimulated to release adrenocorticotropic hormone (ACTH), in addition to altering several other autonomic functions in response to the infection. Finally, there is a dramatic increase in the proliferation of both the T cells and the B cells that have specificity for the pneumococcal organism. All of these changes represent regulation and coordination of multiple organ systems by the immune response to a foreign antigen.

The critical signal molecules that can coordinate these responses are derived directly from the clonal selection of CD4 helper T lymphocytes. Some of the signal molecules (cytokines) are monokines, derived from the antigen-presenting cell (APC), while others are lymphokines, derived from selected CD4 lymphocytes. Production of all the cytokines is critically dependent on the formation of a unique trimolecular complex (class II major histocompatibility complex [MHC] molecule–processed antigen fragment–T-cell receptor) and the subsequent clonal selection of a helper T cell. Fig. 6-1 summarizes many of the activities of the cytokines introduced in this chapter and stresses that the response to an antigen requires activities in several organ systems, which are coordinated by cytokines derived from the immune response.

FUNCTIONS OF INTERLEUKIN-2: T-CELL GROWTH FACTOR

Clonal selection of the CD4 helper T lymphocyte is a decisive event necessary for the successful induction of an immune response. This process of clonal selection has been discussed many times in previous chapters. What has not been discussed in much detail are the events immediately following selection of a specific CD4 T lymphocyte. Both the selected T lymphocyte and the APC are stimulated to produce cytokines. Cytokines from both cells are required for the subsequent T-cell proliferation that must take place to generate a response of sufficient magnitude. In addition, immunologic memory and coordination of inflammatory activities of other tissues sites are dependent on these cytokines.

The proliferation of selected T lymphocytes requires Interleukin-2 (IL-2), a cytokine with T-cell growth factor activity. The IL-2, however, is synthesized and released by the selected CD4 T-cell; that is, the cell that requires the growth factor makes and secretes the necessary factor. IL-2 is, then, a cytokine with an autocrine mode of action. A summary of the initial CD4 T-cell response upon clonal selection is outlined in Fig. 6-2.

In order to proliferate in response to the antigen, the T cell must be stimulated by the IL-2 it synthesized. However, the selected CD4 T lymphocyte normally expresses a low-affinity receptor for the IL-2 molecule and, therefore, cannot respond to low concentrations of the IL-2 signal. Consequently, T-cell proliferation does not take place. Therefore clonal selection of the specific T lymphocyte, by itself, is insufficient to start the events in the immune response.

Signaling Motifs
Autocrine: *The cytokine is produced by the cell that eventually uses the signal molecule.*
Paracrine: *A cell produces a cytokine that is used by one of its neighboring cells.*
Endocrine: *The cell producing this cytokine is at a significant distance from the target of the cytokine action, requiring its transportation through the circulatory system to its site of action.*

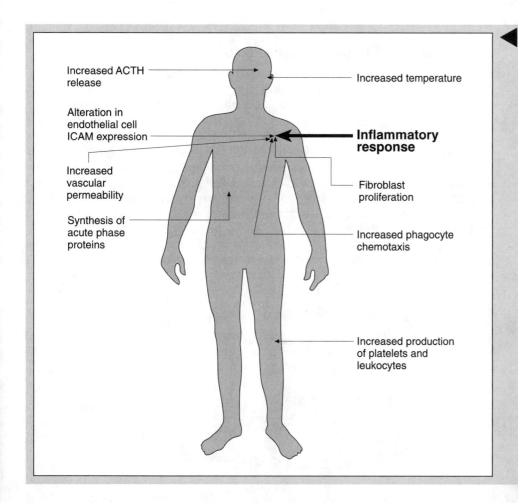

FIGURE 6-1
Spectrum of Biologic Activities Associated with Inflammatory Response. *In the clinical scenario, the infecting organism localizes in the lungs and the draining lymph nodes. However, the immune response to the stimulation of the immune system involves multiple locations, tissues, and organ systems. It is important to understand that all of the changes that take place in response to an inflammatory challenge are the direct result of immune system activation. Following clonal selection of CD4 helper T lymphocytes, cytokines released by both the selected CD4 lymphocyte and the antigen-presenting cell exhibit potent paracrine, autocrine, and endocrine activities, which are responsible for organizing the coordinated responses. ACTH = adrenocorticotropic hormone; ICAM = intercellular adhesion molecules.*

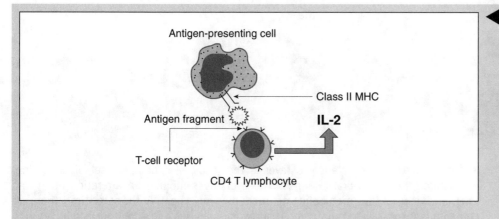

FIGURE 6-2
Initial Events upon Selection of a CD4 Lymphocyte. *Upon clonal selection of an antigen-specific CD4 T lymphocyte, a complex is formed between the class II MHC molecule on the antigen-presenting cell (APC), the processed antigen fragment, and the antigen-specific T-cell receptor. This critical event in the immune response stimulates both the CD4 lymphocyte and the APC. To respond successfully to the antigen challenge, the CD4 lymphocyte must proliferate. The cytokine signal having the T-cell growth-factor activity is a cytokine called interleukin-2 (IL-2), which is synthesized by the selected CD4 lymphocyte. However, the selected CD4 lymphocyte possesses only a low-affinity cell-surface receptor for the IL-2 molecule, consequently the IL-2 signal is ineffective in stimulating proliferation of the selected CD4 lymphocyte.*

MONOKINES

The factors produced by stimulated monocytes, other APCs, and monokines include a rich array of important regulatory molecules that influence many aspects of the immune response.

Interleukin-1 and Tumor Necrosis Factor

Costimulatory Activity for IL-2. During clonal selection of the CD4 T lymphocyte, the APC is also stimulated. One of the early cytokines produced in this response is tumor necrosis factor (TNF), which has a variety of activities. A major activity is an autocrine function, in which the TNF stimulates APCs to produce interleukin-1 (IL-1). IL-1 and TNF have multiple and similar paracrine, autocrine, and endocrine activities. One of the activities for the TNF and IL-1 set of monokines is to stimulate directly the clonally selected T lymphocyte. IL-1 stimulation induces the selected T lymphocyte to produce a polypeptide chain that increases the CD4 cell's affinity for IL-2. Consequently, in the presence of IL-1, the IL-2 produced by the selected T lymphocyte can now bind to the high-affinity receptor and provide the growth factor signal necessary for T-cell proliferation. This relationship between IL-1 and IL-2 in the clonal selection and the activation of helper T lymphocytes is illustrated in Fig. 6-3. If either the antigen-specific clonal selection of the T cell or the IL-1 signal that increases the receptor affinity for IL-2 is missing, there will be no immune response.

FIGURE 6-3 ▶

Stimulation of CD4 Lymphocytes Requires Coexpression of Interleukin-1 (IL-1). *Upon selection of the appropriate CD4 lymphocyte, both the CD4 lymphocyte and the antigen-presenting cell (APC) are stimulated. The stimulated APC begins to secrete tumor necrosis factor and eventually IL-1. IL-1 has multiple activities, and one early activity is to stimulate the selected CD4 lymphocyte to produce an additional polypeptide chain for the CD4 cell's receptor for interleukin-2 (IL-2). This IL-1–dependent modification of the IL-2 receptor increases the affinity of the IL-2 receptor for the IL-2 that is being synthesized by the CD4 cell, and it permits the IL-2 molecule to stimulate CD4 cell proliferation. IL-2 acts as an autocrine signal in the regulation of CD4-lymphocyte proliferation. In this situation, only the CD4 lymphocytes that have been selected by an appropriate class II MHC–antigen complex and have received the IL-1 signal from an activated APC will be allowed to proliferate in response to the antigen.*

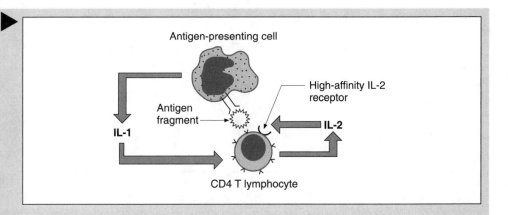

Antigen-presenting cell

High-affinity IL-2 receptor

Antigen fragment

IL-1

IL-2

CD4 T lymphocyte

Thermoregulation. Mrs. Neilson's fever is the result of a complex set of endocrine, autonomic, and behavioral changes. These changes include an alteration of thyroid function to increase the metabolic rate, producing more heat. At the same time, there are autonomic changes in the diameter of surface capillaries and an autonomic increase in the activity of the sweat glands. In addition, there are changes in Mrs. Neilson's behavior. She becomes more lethargic and experiences loss of appetite. All of these endocrine, autonomic, and behavioral processes are responses to IL-1 and TNF.

The change in Mrs. Neilson's temperature can be considered a part of her natural immune response to the pneumococcal organism. The elevated temperature decreases the efficiency of bacterial reproduction while increasing the activity of her lymphocyte responses to the microorganism.

Alteration of Endothelial Cell Surfaces. In a paracrine regulatory motif, IL-1 causes local endothelial cells to increase synthesis and expression of intracellular adhesion molecules (ICAMs). Consequently, circulating neutrophils, when stimulated to express their cell-adhesion molecules (integrins), interact with endothelial cells near an inflammatory site. The neutrophils leave the rapidly flowing blood and, under the influence of chemotactic factors, migrate to the site of the inflammation.

Pyrogens
Several different bacteria contain, in their cell wall, lipopolysaccharide molecules called pyrogens, or exogenous pyrogens. These molecules act directly on tissue histiocytes (macrophages) to stimulate their production of endogenous pyrogen, or IL-1.

Acute Phase Response. Mrs. Neilson's physician found that her ESR was elevated. This is another response to the IL-1 and TNF signals. These inflammatory cytokines act in an endocrine manner directly on the liver to stimulate acute phase protein synthesis. In addition, in an autocrine motif, IL-1 stimulates APCs to induce the synthesis of interleukin-6 (IL-6). IL-6 is a cytokine with multiple functions, one of which is an endocrine-like activity on the liver, resulting in the acute phase response.

The above activities of IL-1 and TNF are summarized in Fig. 6-4. Continued study of immunology will reveal more activities and functions associated with this set of cytokines. However, the activities outlined above are critical to understanding how the immune response happens, and how it coordinates activities of other organ systems. It should be noted that, although the stimulated APC is a major source of IL-1 and TNF, there are also other cells and tissues capable of producing this molecule.

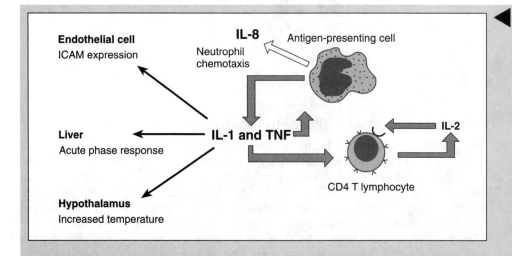

FIGURE 6-4
Autocrine, Endocrine, and Paracrine Activities of Interleukin-1 (IL-1) and Tumor Necrosis Factor (TNF). The IL-1 and TNF set of cytokines have multiple activities directed at several different target tissues. In an autocrine motif, the IL-1 and TNF set of cytokines stimulates the antigen-presenting cell (APC), further activating many of the cell's functions, including the synthesis and release of additional cytokines. One of the IL-1- and TNF-dependent cytokines is interleukin-8 (IL-8), a monokine with potent neutrophil chemotactic activity. In a paracrine motif, the IL-1 and TNF set of cytokines stimulates the selected CD4 lymphocyte as well as local endothelial cells to increase the expression of their intercellular adhesion molecules (ICAMs). In an endocrine motif, the IL-1 and TNF set of cytokines stimulates several different organ systems, such as the hypothalamus, to affect temperature and other autonomic responses, and the liver, to stimulate the acute phase response.

Neutrophil Chemotactic Activity: Interleukin-8

A specimen from Mrs. Neilson's lungs would reveal alveoli that were filled with neutrophils. The effect that IL-1 has on the surface of the local endothelial cells cannot, by itself, explain how the neutrophils are able to migrate selectively toward the site of her inflammation. This directed migration is under the control of another critical monokine, interleukin-8 (IL-8). IL-8, synthesized by the stimulated APC, is a potent chemotactic factor for the neutrophil. Neutrophils binding to capillary endothelial cells detect IL-8 and migrate to the source of the chemotactic factor, that is, to the site of inflammation. This functional relationship between the APC, endothelial cell, and neutrophil is schematically illustrated in Fig. 6-5. This figure demonstrates again how the immune response is capable of coordinating the functional activities of several tissues.

Cell Growth and Repair Factors

Repair Cytokines. During the course of any inflammatory response, there is tissue damage associated with the initial injury, colonization by an invading microorganism, or an immune response to the antigen (hypersensitivity reaction). Local somatic cells need to be induced to proliferate in an attempt to repair the damaged tissues. It is the APC that again produces the necessary growth and differentiation factors allowing these repair processes to take place. These growth factors are named according to the cells they affect. A partial list includes fibroblast growth factor (FGF), platelet-derived growth factor (PDGF), and transforming growth factor β (TGF-β).

*Platelets were the first identified source of **platelet-derived growth factor**. The identical molecule is also synthesized by activated APCs.*

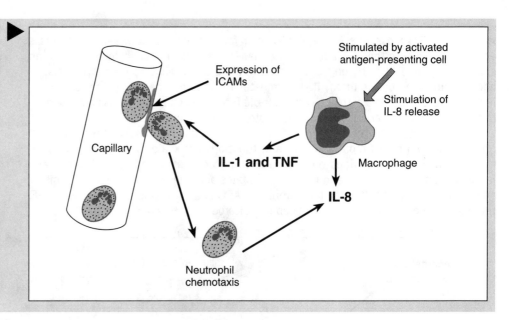

Hematopoietic Stem Cell Growth Factors

Stimulation of Leukopoiesis. In any inflammatory reaction, there is a significant amount of leukocyte death. As discussed above, a vast number of neutrophils are recruited to the inflammatory tissues. Upon stimulation at the inflammatory site, these cells are activated, carry out their function, and then die. Similarly, lymphocytes and monocytes are recruited to the inflamed tissues, and many of these cells are destroyed by the release of toxic molecules at the inflammatory site. To maintain adequate numbers of leukocytes for a sustained response to the current infection or for future infections, the bone marrow must receive signals to increase the production of the types of cells that are being consumed. These signals come in the form of growth and differentiation factors for bone marrow–derived stem cells. There are specific factors that stimulate the growth and differentiation for the lineage of each leukocyte. For example, granulocyte colony-stimulating factor (G-CSF) provides the information for stem cell–derived granulocyte precursors to continue growing, differentiating, and forming granulocytes. Similarly, granulocyte-monocyte colony-stimulating factor (GM-CSF) promotes the development of both granulocytes and monocytes from the bone marrow pluripotent stem cell.

Table 6-2 provides a summary of those monokines that are critical to understanding the immune system and, in many cases, how immune responses control the activities of other tissue types. It is important to remember that, like the other cytokines, the monocyte is not the sole cellular source for these factors. Moreover, the monokines have cofactor or costimulatory activities for many other cell types not discussed here.

TABLE 6-2 ▶

Monokines

Monokine	Activity
IL-1 and TNF	Inflammatory: induction of monocyte–cytokine synthesis, expression of CAMs, induction of fever, and stimulation of acute phase response
IL-8	Neutrophil chemotactic factor
IL-6	Acute phase response; leukocyte growth and differentiation
GM-CSF (and other CSFs)	Granulocyte-monocyte colony-stimulating factor Cytotoxic factors
Growth factors (TGF-β, PDGF, FGF)	Activation and growth regulation; tissue repair

Note. ICAMs = intracellular cell adhesion molecules; IL = interleukin; TNF = tumor necrosis factor; GM-CSF = granulocyte-monocyte colony-stimulating factor; TGF-β = transforming growth factor β; PDGF = platelet-derived growth factor; FGF = fibroblast growth factor.

LYMPHOKINES

Helper T-Cell Factors

IL-2 is not the sole lymphokine produced in response to clonal selection. Activated helper T (Th) cells also make a variety of products that mediate Th1 and Th2 cell functions. These products of Th1 and Th2 cells were discussed in Chap. 5. Briefly, Th2 cells produce the IL-4, IL-5, and IL-6, which allow B cells to proliferate, switch isotypes, and differentiate into antibody-secreting plasma cells or memory cells. Th1 cells, on the other hand, produce IL-2 for the growth of both CD4 and CD8 T lymphocytes, and they produce interferon-γ (IFN-γ), which mediates delayed-type hypersensitivity (DTH) reactions.

Hematopoietic Stem Cell Growth Factor: Interleukin-3

In addition to the cytokines that mediate Th1 and Th2 activities, CD4 cells produce leukocyte growth and differentiation factors. One of the most conspicuous of these lymphokines is interleukin-3 (IL-3). IL-3 has a panhematopoietic stem cell growth factor activity and can augment the development of all hematopoietic cells. In addition, GM-CSF and G-CSF are synthesized by the selected CD4 lymphocyte. Table 6-3 lists the major lymphokines produced by the selected CD4 cell populations.

◀ ***TABLE 6-3***
Lymphokines

Cytokines	Th1 Cells	Th2 Cells
IL-3 (hematopoietic growth factor)	+	+
GM-CSF (granulocyte-monocyte colony-stimulating factor)	+	+
IL-2 (T cell growth factor)	+	−
IFN-γ (delayed-type hypersensitivity)	+	−
IL-4	−	+
IL-5	−	+
IL-6	−	+
IL-10	−	+

Note. Th = helper T (cell); IL = interleukin; IFN-γ = interferon-γ.

INTERACTIONS BETWEEN THE IMMUNE SYSTEM AND OTHER REGULATORY SYSTEMS

In Chap. 1, the immune system was likened to the central and autonomic nervous systems, because the systems are capable of modifying the responses of other tissues and organs. These regulatory systems also interact with each other. The interactions are complex, and the complexity is compounded by the lack of knowledge in this rapidly growing and changing field. Mrs. Neilson's fever response provides an excellent indication of how the immune system can interfere with the autonomic nervous system. However, the best example of the interactions and mutual regulation between the immune system and other regulatory systems is probably the relationship between the immune system and adrenal function (Fig. 6-6). Mrs. Neilson is experiencing a massive production of IL-1. One of the functions of the lymphokine is to stimulate the hypothalamus, which, in addition to altering body temperature, promotes the secretion of ACTH. The elevated ACTH levels stimulate increased production of cortical steroids by the adrenals. These steroids include molecules, such as cortisol, that have potent anti-inflammatory activity and can suppress further immunologic function. Consequently, a

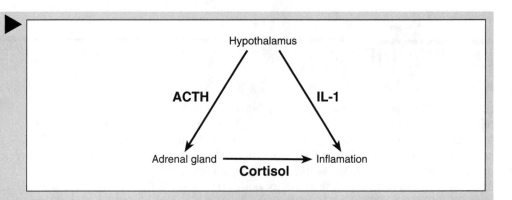

FIGURE 6-6

Connections between Endocrine System, Autonomic Nervous System, and Immune System. *The endocrine system, autonomic nervous system, and immune system are connected and have integrated methods of control. These control mechanisms are not clearly defined. One of the more obvious connections between the systems relates to the connection between inflammation and the synthesis of stress hormones. Interleukin-1 (IL-1), released in response to an antigen challenge, increases the production of glucocorticoids through the hypothalamus–pituitary–adrenal axis. The resulting cortisol production suppresses responses of the inflammatory cells. ACTH = adrenocorticotropic hormone.*

temporary generalized suppression of the immune response would not be unexpected as a result of the above interactions. It must be stressed, however, that this is but one example of the connections between the immune system and other regulatory systems.

Superantigens

Several organisms, including some viruses and the bacteria responsible for toxic shock syndrome, as well as some types of food poisoning, produce a bifunctional molecule. This molecule, called a superantigen, has a binding site for the common component of the T-cell receptor. Consequently, it binds to all T cells, regardless of the antigen-binding specificity. The second site on the superantigen binds to a common structure on all class II MHC molecules, creating a molecule that can effectively mimic the trimolecular complex necessary for clonal selection of CD4 lymphocytes, with one important exception: there is no antigen specificity associated with the clonal selection. Therefore, all CD4 cells and monocytes bound by the superantigen begin producing all of their inflammatory products. The massive cytokine production at multiple locations prevents cytokine gradients from being established, and there can be no coordinated response to a single location. The net result is, essentially, a paralysis of the immune system and immunosuppression.

RESOLUTION OF CLINICAL CASE

One week prior to Mrs. Neilson's visit to the emergency room, she experienced an upper respiratory viral infection. The virus infected the epithelial cells lining her bronchial tree and eventually induced a cell-mediated response to the virus. Both the virus and the immune response to the virus damaged the cilia that help prevent access of organisms to the lungs (natural immunity), putting Mrs. Neilson at risk for a secondary infection.

Mrs. Neilson, unfortunately, contracted a pneumococcal infection. The immune response to the organism eventually resulted in antibody synthesis and a humoral immune response. Fig. 6-7 provides a global summary of the roles of cytokines in these reactions.

Antibody-opsonized organisms (in addition to bacterial cell wall components) stimulated the monocytes to produce and secrete monokines. The TNF and IL-1, initially secreted by the macrophages, have a spectrum of activities on multiple target organs (Fig. 6-7). The patient's temperature increased, she began synthesizing acute phase proteins, her behaviors changed, and the endothelial cells lining the capillaries of the lungs began synthesizing and expressing increased amounts of ICAMs. Moreover, the proportions of the different cell types synthesized in the bone marrow changed. Monocytes in the area of the inflammatory response also synthesized and secreted IL-8, a factor that is chemotactic for neutrophils, and helped direct the neutrophils to the site of

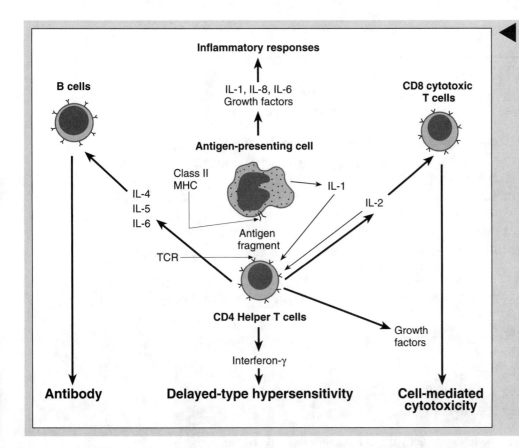

◄ *FIGURE 6-7*
Central Role of CD4 Lymphocytes in the Immune Response. Formation of a trimolecular complex between the class II MHC molecules on the antigen-presenting cell (APC), the processed antigen fragment, and the T-cell receptor initiates a cascade of events that are central to immune responses. These events are under the direction of the cytokines released from both the selected CD4 lymphocyte and the APC. Monokines released from the APC coordinate the inflammatory responses of multiple organ systems. Cytokines released from the CD4 Th2 cell can permit selected B lymphocytes to proliferate, switch isotype, and differentiate into either plasma cells or memory cells. Cytokines released from the CD4 Th1 cells can provide help for cytotoxic T lymphocytes and mediate the cellular responses of the delayed-type hypersensitivity (DTH) reaction. CD4 cytokines can also stimulate increased leukopoiesis in the bone marrow. IL = interleukin; Th = T helper.

the inflammatory response. As a result of the cellular infiltrate and cytotoxic activities of the activated cells, Mrs. Neilson's lungs began filling with fluid and blood and then with activated neutrophils and monocytes, which actively engaged in the destruction of the microorganism. The activities of the immune system, along with responses from several organ systems, provided Mrs. Neilson with a coordinated method to protect herself against the bacterial infection. These immune and organ system responses successfully prevented further colonization. However, much of the pathology (i.e., hypersensitivity) experienced by Mrs. Neilson resulted from the response of the immune system itself.

REVIEW QUESTIONS

Directions: For each of the following questions, choose the **one best** answer.

1. Which of the following statements about cytokines is correct?

   (A) Each of the cytokines responsible for inflammatory reactions has a unique cell source.

   (B) Each of the cytokines responsible for inflammatory reactions has a single target tissue.

   (C) One cytokine cannot modify the reactions of another cytokine.

   (D) Although there are differences in concentration, different cell types can produce the same cytokine.

2. Which of the following cytokines is necessary for the proliferation of antigen-selected CD4 T lymphocytes?

   (A) IL-1

   (B) IL-2

   (C) IL-8

   (D) IL-1 and IL-2

   (E) IL-1, IL-2, and IL-8

3. Which of the following activities is associated with IL-1 and TNF?

   (A) Stimulation of a high-affinity receptor for IL-2 on selected CD4 lymphocytes

   (B) Suppression of macrophage activation and cytokine secretion

   (C) Inhibition of acute phase protein synthesis by the liver

   (D) Chemotactic factor for neutrophils

4. Which of the following is a correct statement about CD4 cells?

   (A) When a CD4 cell is selected, it begins making all of the cytokines associated with both Th1 and Th2 cells.

   (B) When the CD4 cell is selected, it begins making the cytokines associated with the Th1-type reactions. However, with time, the cell switches to making the cytokines associated with the Th2-type reactions.

   (C) The mechanism by which a selected CD4 cell starts making the Th1 or Th2 pattern of cytokines is not currently understood.

   (D) Once a CD4 cell has been selected, it differentiates, such that Th1 and Th2 cells can be clearly distinguished by the use of cell-surface markers.

5. Repair of damaged tissues is also a consequence of the inflammatory reaction. Which of the following cells is the primary source of tissue repair factors?

   (A) Macrophages

   (B) CD8 lymphocytes

   (C) CD4 lymphocytes

   (D) Neutrophils

Note. Abbreviations used in the questions: IL = interleukin; Th1 and Th2 = helper T-1 and T-2 cells; FGF = fibroblast growth factor; TGF = transforming growth factor; PDGF = platelet-derived growth factor; GM–CSF = granulocyte-monocyte colony-stimulating factor; INF-γ = interferon-γ; G-CSF = granulocyte colony-stimulating factor.

6. Which of the following factors is primarily responsible for replacing neutrophils that have been consumed as the result of an inflammatory response?

    (A) IL-2

    (B) GM-CSF

    (C) FGF

    (D) IL-8

    (E) INF-γ

7. Which of the following CD4 lymphokines has a growth factor activity for several hematopoietic cell types?

    (A) IL-1

    (B) IL-2

    (C) IL-3

    (D) IL-8

    (E) IFN-γ

8. An isolated T lymphocyte was found to produce large amounts of IL-10. Which of the following cell populations is most probably associated with this cell?

    (A) CD8 lymphocytes

    (B) Cytotoxic T lymphocytes

    (C) CD4 Th1 lymphocytes

    (D) CD4 Th2 lymphocytes

ANSWERS AND EXPLANATIONS

1. **The answer is D.** Multiple cell types can produce the same cytokine, however, there may be significant differences in concentration. Similarly, a single cytokine may have slightly different functions on different target tissues. Moreover, many cytokines exhibit costimulatory activity, in which one cytokine can modify the activity of another cytokine.

2. **The answer is D.** Although IL-2, has a T-cell growth factor activity, IL-1 is necessary to induce the production of a high-affinity IL-2 receptor on the surface of the CD4 lymphocyte.

3. **The answer is A.** IL-1 and TNF have autocrine, endocrine, and paracrine activities that activate many phases of the inflammatory response. IL-8, however, has potent neutrophil chemotactic activity.

4. **The answer is C.** Both CD4 and the Th1 and Th2 cells appear to be selected similarly. It is, however, not clear how subsequent events take place to generate either the Th1-type or Th2-type of helper cells.

5. **The answer is A.** Factors such as FGF, TGF, and PDGF are monokines and are responsible for the repair of tissues damaged as a result of an injury or an inflammatory response.

6. **The answer is B.** G-CSF and GM-CSF are produced by macrophages, and they promote the development of granulocytes from the bone marrow–derived stem cell.

7. **The answer is C.** IL-3, an endocrine-like molecule released by selected CD4 cells, stimulates a general hematopoiesis in the bone marrow.

8. **The answer is D.** IL-10 is a cytokine associated with CD4 Th2 cell function. The cytokine prevents the synthesis of CD4 Th1 cytokines; thus, it is thought to have an important regulatory activity.

PART II: LEARNING ISSUES

7 ANTIGENS, IMMUNOGENS, AND AUTOANTIGENS

CHAPTER OUTLINE

INTRODUCTION OF CLINICAL CASE

Mrs. Schwartz, a 56-year-old woman, consulted her physician, complaining of increasing lethargy and malaise. She reported stiff and painful joints, which were most bothersome in the mornings. She

Given the information in the laboratory findings, what would Mrs. Schwartz's serum levels of interleukin-1 (IL-1) be, compared to the normal values?

could identify no unique time, event, or activity that coincided with the onset of her symptoms. Physical examination revealed signs of inflammation in the joints of her hands and feet. An x-ray of the affected hand joints showed a narrowing of the articular cartilage and alterations in normal joint structure. Laboratory investigations demonstrated an increased erythrocyte sedimentation rate (ESR), a decrease in serum complement levels, a negative serum antibody test for Lyme disease, and the presence of immunoglobulin M (IgM) antibody in her blood, which specifically agglutinates particles coated with human immunoglobulin. Analysis of the synovial fluid showed no bacteria or crystals; however, a significant number of neutrophils was found.

FACTORS THAT INFLUENCE IMMUNOGENICITY

In Mrs. Schwartz, the presence of IgM antibody, which can agglutinate human immunoglobulin-coated particles, shows that her immunoglobulin molecules are themselves antigens or, more correctly, autoantigens. Mrs. Schwartz is immunologically responding to her own immunoglobulin molecules. This finding raises questions about how to define antigens. Clearly, in this case, the characteristic of being foreign is, alone, an insufficient criterion for determining what is and what is not an antigen.

When discussing antigen characteristics, it is important to distinguish between materials that simply bind to antibody and those that induce a new immune response. Generally, the term *immunogen* refers to materials that induce an immune response, and the term *antigen* implies reaction with or binding to antibody or a T cell. This distinction is not fixed, however, and the terms are often used interchangeably. Using this definition, an antigen need not have all the physical or chemical properties necessary to induce an immune response. Immunogens are antigens, but the reverse is not necessarily true. Immunogens have some basic properties, including foreignness, molecular size, chemical composition, digestibility, host genetics, and dose and route of exposure that confers the ability to induce an immune response.

Foreignness

Foreignness is usually the first item mentioned in any discussion of what makes something immunogenic. Clearly, foreign molecules can be immunogenic; however, as we have seen in the above case, this criterion alone will not prevent self-structures from inducing an immune response. Autoimmunity can be viewed both as positive and negative. The ability of self-components to elicit an immune response is important for the removal of dying or injured cells, as well as for the removal of inactivated or modified macromolecular self-structures. Only when this anti-self-response is out of control and there is accompanying pathology, as in Mrs. Schwartz's case, is the anti-self-response considered disease. Apparently, everyone has autoreactive B and T lymphocytes, and the responsiveness of these cells is usually well controlled.

Molecular Size

Size is a second important criterion that helps determine if a molecule is an immunogen. However, like the concept of foreignness, size alone is insufficient to induce an immune response. Molecules below a certain size do not, by themselves, induce an immune response because they are missing some of the other essential characteristics of immunogens. The immune system, however, can be fooled into responding to small molecules. Such molecules are *haptens*. In order for haptens to induce an immune response, they need to be coupled to larger carrier molecules that confer to the hapten the other characteristics of immunogens. In this relationship between haptens and carriers, the hapten can convey one of the characteristics for immunogenicity (i.e., foreignness), while the carrier confers the other immunogenicity-determining factors to the hapten (Fig. 7-1).

A complex protein molecule can be thought of as a series of haptens that are all connected to a common carrier. In this case, the individual hapten-like components of the macromolecule are called *epitopes* (Fig. 7-2).

Chemical Composition

Diversity in chemical composition of a molecule is a third characteristic that leads to increased immunogenicity. A macromolecule that exhibits all of the other factors influencing immunogenicity, but exhibits only one or a small number of epitopes, can clonally select only a limited number of T or B cells. On the other hand, if that same macromolecule expresses many different epitopes, there is a greater probability for that heterogeneous structure clonally to select a T or B cell.

Digestibility

One critical difference between the molecules that are antigens and those that can induce an immune response relates to whether or not they can be chemically fragmented by the processing mechanisms of the antigen-presenting cells (APCs). As has been previously stressed, an effective secondary immune response requires the chemical alteration of a sample of the antigen for presentation by the class I or class II major histocompatibility complex (MHC) molecule. If a molecule cannot be processed by APCs

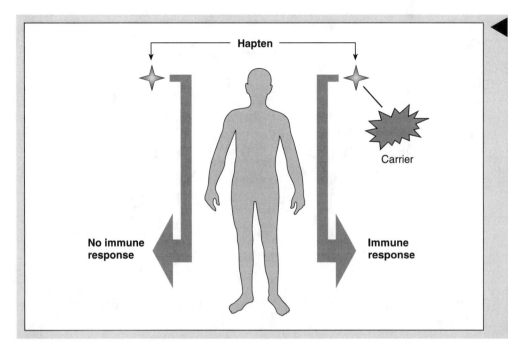

FIGURE 7-1
Hapten Carrier Response. When an individual is immunized with a hapten or a single antigenic site, there is no immune response. However, if the hapten is covalently coupled with a protein that possesses the other immunogenicity determining factors, such as larger molecular size, chemical complexity, and the ability to be hydrolyzed by the cellular-processing machinery, there is an immune response not only to the carrier but also to the hapten, or single epitope. Using hapten carrier complexes, it is possible to prepare antibody that is specific for small organic molecules that would not normally induce an immune response.

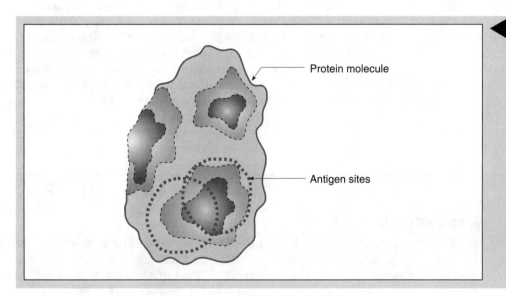

FIGURE 7-2
Epitope Structure of Proteins. Proteins can be viewed as a collection of several protein-surface epitopes (individual antigenic sites). Collectively, these epitopes cover most of the surface of a protein but are most prominent on the more exposed surfaces. Although antibodies from different clones of B lymphocytes can be directed to the same epitope, these antibodies may react with overlapping areas of the antigen surface, as depicted by the dashed line in this figure.

or expressed on the cell surface in association with the MHC molecules, then there is no secondary immune response. The ability to be altered by the processing enzymes and by digestibility is the fourth critical characteristic for the carrier component of immunogens.

Host Genetics

The genetic constitution of the host also plays a central role in immune responsiveness. Although there are multiple genetic factors that can influence immune responses, the role of the MHC molecules in presenting antigen is clear. The MHC molecules express tremendous diversity, some of which is found in the peptide-binding site. Different MHC molecules would be expected to hold the same processed antigen differently or, possibly, not at all. Consequently, the nature of the subsequent immune response would be different (Fig. 7-3).

The genetic component of immunogenicity is linked to several diseases. If a particular MHC molecule holds a processed antigen in a conformation that resembles a normal self-structure, there is the real possibility that infection with or exposure to that

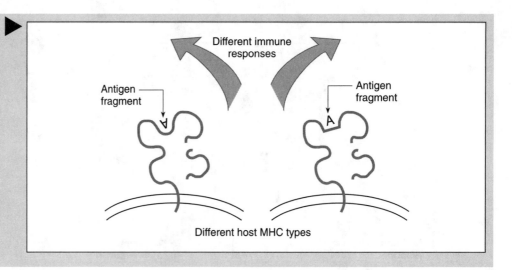

agent may adversely effect the normal immune regulation to that cross-reactive self-component.

Dose and Route

Equally important to all of the above items that characterize immunogens is the way in which the host initially encounters the immunizing agent. Both the route of exposure as well as the amount of antigen are of critical importance in determining the type and nature of the eventual immune response. For each antigen, there is a critical concentration that is necessary to induce an immune response. This is easily understood by remembering that, to induce an immune response, the antigen must physically interact with the appropriate B lymphocyte and be presented to the appropriate CD4 T lymphocyte.

ANTIGEN TYPES

Simple Antigens

Biologic macromolecules are simple antigens that can be viewed as assemblies of smaller molecular-weight components connected by hydrolyzable linkages. Fig. 7-4 illustrates a schematic structure of a protein antigen. The surface structure of the protein represents the collection of different epitopes or antigenic sites that can bind to either antibody or the B-cell receptor for antigen. These antigenic sites cover the entire surface of the protein or macromolecule. Amino acid substitutions, when expressed on the surface, alter the reaction with antibody and, potentially, induce a totally new immune response. Similarly, changes in the three-dimensional structure of the epitopes alter the interaction with antibody. If one of these sites could be dissected from the intact antigen while maintaining its unique three-dimensional structure, it would continue to react with the relevant antibody. This property provides an important tool that can be used to analyze the structure of another protein and induces antibody responses to both the synthetic peptide and the model-protein molecule. From this discussion, it should become obvious that B-cell antigens exhibit a critical three-dimensional conformation component. Altering the conformation dramatically alters the reaction with antibody.

Simple antigens also stimulate T lymphocytes. However, in the case of T-cell antigens, the characteristics are very different from the B-cell antigen. This difference is the direct result of the antigen processing and MHC binding of the processed antigen (Fig. 7-5). The processing requirement for a T-cell response implies that, instead of the conformational antigenic structures seen with B-cell antigens, T-cell antigens represent a sequential structure along the polymer chain. Therefore, T-cell antigenic sites include

*B-cell antigens have a major **conformational** component. T-cell antigens are **sequential** in nature and represent linear sequences of the parent biologic molecule.*

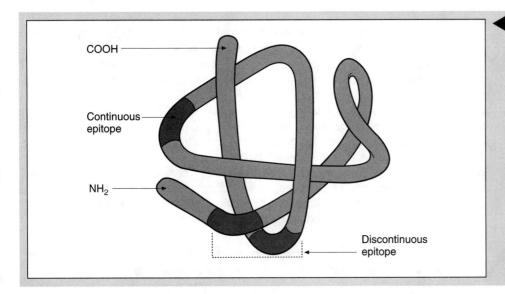

◀ **FIGURE 7-4**
Model of B-Cell Antigen. *B cells are selected by directly binding the antigen, which results in B-cell antigens exhibiting a significant three-dimensional component. Antigenic sites, therefore, represent the original configuration of the antigen molecule. For example, if a linear sequence of a protein molecule is exposed on the surface, then the entire continuous amino acid region may be part of a protein epitope. On the other hand, if two amino acid sequences from different parts of the same molecule are associated on the protein surface, this set of discontinuous sequences will be part of the same protein epitope. Protein epitopes for B lymphocytes are three-dimensional and may be either continuous or discontinuous. COOH = carboxyl terminal; NH_2 = amino terminal.*

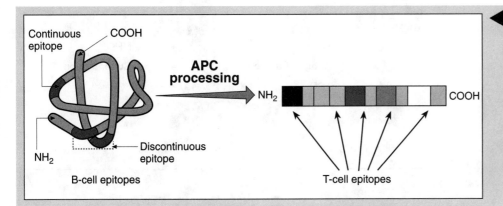

◀ **FIGURE 7-5**
Model of T-Cell Antigen. *T-cell antigens are different from B-cell antigens because of the processing requirements for T lymphocytes. During the processing events, the three-dimensional nature of the B-cell antigen is destroyed, and a series of linear peptide sequences are produced. These linear sequences are held by the major histocompatibility complex molecules and presented to T lymphocytes. COOH = carboxyl terminal; NH_2 = amino terminal.*

not only peptide fragments from the exterior of the molecule but also peptide fragments from the core of the molecule that have not been exposed to solvent. In considering differences between T- and B-cell antigens, it should be remembered that biologic molecules can be denatured and partially degraded prior to electing a B-cell response, and thus it is possible to obtain antibodies to a denatured form of a molecule. Generally speaking, antibodies to native molecules do not cross-react with antibodies to denatured molecules, and vice versa.

Mitogens. There are some unique biologic molecules that are often considered antigens because they can stimulate cells of the immune system via different mechanisms. One of these unique antigens is the mitogen. Mitogens include plant proteins, such as concanavalin A or pokeweed mitogen, as well as other molecules that can induce mitosis. Two common characteristics of the mitogens are that they either possess multiple binding sites for carbohydrate residues expressed on cell surfaces, including T and B lymphocytes, or they perturb cell membranes. When the mitogen binds to and cross-links the target cell-surface structures, the target cell is stimulated to undergo mitosis. In this respect, the mitogen stimulates a variety of cellular processes in addition to mitotic events and mimics the effect of antigen. A major difference between mitogen and antigen stimulation of lymphocytes is that, with mitogens, no associated antigenic specificity (i.e., a polyclonal response) is observed upon mitogen stimulation, whereas antigen stimulation selects only specific B or T cells.

One application of the mitogen response is in the investigation of the responsiveness of the immune system. The complete blood cell (CBC) count evaluates only the numbers of cells present in the clinical sample. This cell count, however, tells little about the responsiveness of the cell populations that were counted. Mitogens, on the other hand, can be used, in part, to determine whether or not the cells that were counted are able to respond to stimulation.

Superantigen. A second type of special "antigen" is the superantigen. Superantigens more closely mimic the activities of more conventional antigens in that they stimulate the formation of a trimolecular complex between T cells and APCs. Consequently, both the T cell and the APC are stimulated to produce inflammatory cytokines. Superantigens accomplish this because they contain two different binding sites on a single molecule. One of these sites binds to a location that is common to all T-cell receptors, whereas the second binding site is for the MHC molecule. Fig. 7-6 illustrates the differences between the trimolecular complexes formed by conventional antigens and those formed by superantigens. The consequences of superantigen exposure is a massive release of lymphokines and monokines. However, with a typical antigen, only specific antigen-reactive T cells and the corresponding APC are stimulated to release cytokines. Some of the organisms responsible for food poisoning and toxic shock syndrome exhibit their pathology because of superantigen stimulation.

FIGURE 7-6 ▶

Comparison of Clonal Selection and Superantigen Selection. *Superantigens are protein molecules, produced by some bacteria and viruses, that mimic the structure and function of a trimolecular complex formed by major histocompatibility complex (MHC)–antigen peptide and the T-cell receptor (TCR). Superantigens have two binding sites. One binding site is for the class II MHC molecule found on the antigen-presenting cells, while the other binding site is for a common structure found outside of the antigen-binding site on the TCR. Whereas antigen selection of CD4 T lymphocytes is limited to only the T cell with the TCR that is appropriate to the MHC–antigen complex, superantigens select all T cells, regardless of the TCR antigenic specificity.*

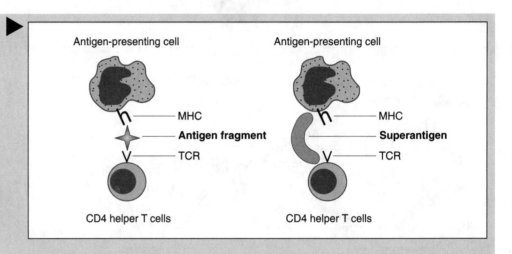

Complex Antigens

Microbial agents provide a source of complex antigens. Complex antigens can be viewed as assemblies of several different macromolecules or simple antigens. Extracellular bacteria provide an antigenic challenge to the immune system with the variety of bacterial structures presented on their cell membranes or cell walls. Bacteria also secrete a variety of proteins and toxins into their environment that also fit the requirements of immunogens. All of these bacterial components can induce antibody and CD4 T lymphocyte responses.

Viruses also induce immune responses. When viruses are extracellular, they are capable of inducing the same types of immune responses as any extracellular complex antigen. However, when sequestered within a cell, the virus is not available to select B lymphocytes or to be presented by the APCs. In this case, the CD8 component of the immune system is primarily responsible for identification and elimination of the viral antigens. This only happens, however, when the cell is actively engaged in synthesizing viral particles. If viral protein is not being translated, then no antigens are expressed that are associated with MHC, and there is no immune response.

VACCINES

One very practical application of the knowledge of antigen structure and biology is the design and construction of vaccines. Vaccines have made a dramatic impact on health care. Currently, there are two very different categories of immunization (Fig. 7-7). One

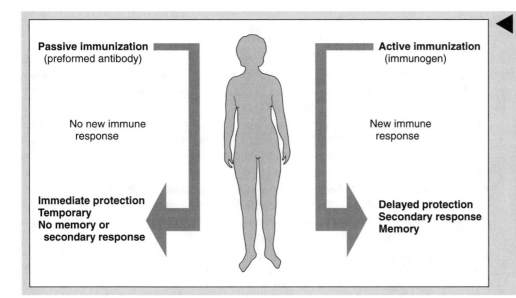

FIGURE 7-7
Effects of Active versus Passive Immunization. *Passive immunization provides an individual with the products of an immune response—antibody (gamma globulin or immune globulin). Passive immunity leads to immediate protection. However, the protection is temporary, and there is no memory response. Active immunization, on the other hand, exposes the individual to the antigen and allows the individual to generate an immune response. With active immunity, protection against the antigen is delayed during the generation of the immune response, but, once the response is established, there is immunologic memory and a secondary immune response.*

type, *passive immunization*, is the administration of the product of an immune response (i.e., antibody). Passive immunization does not activate the immune system, it does not provide memory, and any protection resulting from the administered antibody is lost with the normal biologic turnover of the molecule. The importance of passive immunization is the speed with which immunologic protection can be obtained.

Conversely, in *active immunization* the immune system actively responds to an antigen. Vaccines that induce active immunity and immunologic memory are constructed in many different ways and can contain either simple antigens or complex antigens. Each class of vaccine has its uniquely characteristic immune response, generated length of immunologic memory, and risk-to-benefit ratio of the vaccine. Active vaccines are classified as either a live-organism vaccine (complex antigen) or an inactivated, or partially purified, product from the infectious agent. If the vaccine is a live organism, it must be altered or attenuated to avoid the disease pathology. If the vaccine is composed of a purified product of an infectious agent having a toxic activity, that activity must be removed from the molecule. The altered toxin is termed a *toxoid*.

Nonviable vaccines often need an adjuvant to generate a maximal immune system. For example, protein vaccines for human use are commonly adsorbed onto aluminum phosphate (alum). This alters the route of antigen administration by converting the soluble protein to a particle, which is more easily phagocytized for presentation. In addition, the particulate nature helps direct the antigen to the lymph nodes while preventing a dilution of the immunogen. Some adjuvants also contain components that nonspecifically induce inflammation. Although not used in humans, these adjuvants can have dramatic effects on the magnitude of the subsequent immune response.

Vaccine construction remains an extremely active area of investigation. Current methods of using recombinant proteins, conjugate vaccines, and gene vaccines raise the possibility of using immunization technology to prevent an even broader array of diseases in the future.

*A **toxoid** is a toxin molecule from which the biologic activity has been removed but on which the antigenic sites (epitopes) remain intact. Immunization with a toxoid produces antibody molecules that react with the parent toxin.*

*Purified protein vaccines usually require the use of **adjuvants** to achieve a maximal immune response.*

AUTOANTIGENS

There are multiple hypotheses to account for an altered immune regulation that triggers a continuing autoimmune response. The nature of the event that triggers the response for any particular disease is not clearly understood. In addition to genetic and hormonal involvement, the following five mechanisms are proposed.

Mechanisms for Induction of Autoimmunity

Molecular Mimicry. An agent that, either by itself or in combination with a specific MHC molecule, resembles a self-structure, is an example of molecular mimicry. The subsequent immune response after exposure to the agent cross-reacts with a normal molecule and alters the tolerance to that self-structure.

Alteration of Self-Antigen. A normal self-structure is either chemically altered or modified as a response to some other insult or event. This altered self-structure is now foreign and can induce an immune response that perturbs the regulatory mechanisms for the normal molecule.

Polyclonal Activation of B Cells. Several bacteria and some viruses express or secrete polyclonal activators that nonspecifically activate B or T lymphocytes. If the product of this polyclonal activation reacts with and damages a self-structure, the altered structure may continue to augment the immune response.

Lymphokine Imbalance. Lymphokines play a major role in all aspects of the immune response, including the induction of tolerance. Any event that alters lymphokine levels can have major regulatory effects on the immune system.

Inappropriate MHC Expression or Presentation. There are clearly associations between human leukocyte antigen (HLA) molecules and disease. These associations also exist for autoimmune diseases. It is fairly easy to understand that different MHC molecules can present a common antigen fragment in different conformations. If one of these conformations happens to mimic a self-structure, then there is, again, the potential for an autoimmune response.

RESOLUTION OF CLINICAL CASE

In the clinical scenario, Mrs. Schwartz was responding to a self-antigen. She was making an antibody in response to her own immunoglobulin molecules—an autoantibody or autoimmune response. Autoimmune responses are not uncommon and probably play a major role in the ability of the immune system to survey dead cells, dying cells, or damaged macromolecules routinely. In the case of Mrs. Schwartz, however, something happened to disrupt the normal regulation of the immune response, and the resulting immune response led to the pathology she was experiencing.

REVIEW QUESTIONS

Directions: For each of the following questions, choose the **one best** answer.

1. Which one of the following molecular characteristics defines the minimum set of factors necessary to induce a secondary immune response?

    (A) Foreignness

    (B) Chemical complexity

    (C) Foreignness and chemical complexity

    (D) Foreignness, chemical complexity, and digestibility

2. Which of the following is a correct statement about autoimmune responses?

    (A) Autoimmune responses are always antibody mediated and always associated with significant pathology.

    (B) Autoimmune responses may be either antibody or cell mediated and are always associated with significant pathology.

    (C) Autoimmune responses are always antibody mediated, but detectable pathology may or may not be associated with the response.

    (D) Autoimmune responses may be either antibody or cell mediated, and detectable pathology may or may not be associated with the response.

3. Digestibility, or the ability of a macromolecule to be hydrolized into smaller fragments, reflects which of the following requirements of the antigen?

    (A) It must bind to a B-lymphocyte antigen receptor.

    (B) It must progress through the lymph to a local lymph node.

    (C) It must be processed by an antigen-presenting cell.

    (D) It must interact with antibody.

    (E) It must be cleared from the circulation once it has reacted with an antibody.

4. An adjuvant can increase the immune response to an antigen by which of the following mechanisms?

    (A) Dispersing and solubilizing antigen

    (B) Preventing phagocytosis, so that it can select a B cell

    (C) Directing the antigen to the local lymph nodes

    (D) Maintaining the antigen in peripheral tissues and preventing it from going to the local nodes

5. Which of the following statements about mitogens is correct?

    (A) Mitogens stimulate only T lymphocytes.

    (B) Mitogens stimulate only B lymphocytes.

    (C) Mitogens react with the T-cell receptor and stimulate a monoclonal T-cell response.

    (D) Mitogens react with epithelial cells to induce mitosis.

    (E) Mitogens that react with T lymphocytes can bind to the lymphocyte surface but do not induce mitosis.

6. The generation of which set of the following cytokines would be expected in response to a superantigen exposure?

   (A) Interferon-γ, IL-8 and IL-2

   (B) IL-8 and complement factors

   (C) IL-3, IL-2, and histamine

   (D) IL-1, porins, and IL-2

7. Which of the following is a characteristic of passive immunization?

   (A) Passive immunization does not generate immunologic memory.

   (B) Passive immunization is associated with an isotype switch and secondary immune response.

   (C) Following passive immunization, there is a delay of 12–18 days before the individual is immunologically protected.

   (D) Passive immunity refers only to cell-mediated immunity.

8. An individual has been exposed to a disease-causing organism. Which of the following approaches would best prevent the individual from experiencing disease as a result of exposure?

   (A) No action is necessary because exposure to the organism immunized the individual.

   (B) The individual should be actively immunized with the live organism.

   (C) The individual should be actively immunized with an appropriate vaccine.

   (D) The individual should be passively immunized now and actively immunized later.

9. Which of the following is a correct statement about the induction of an autoimmune response?

   (A) An autoimmune response can only be induced by exposure to a cross-reacting antigen.

   (B) Exposure to an agent that chemically modifies an autologous structure can initiate an autoimmune response.

   (C) There is no genetic component associated with autoimmune responses.

   (D) Abnormal cytokine levels cannot induce autoimmune responses.

ANSWERS AND EXPLANATIONS

1. **The answer is D.** Each of these factors is necessary for the immune response, and each in isolation may give rise to a T-cell–independent response. However, to induce a secondary immune response it is necessary to process (digest) the antigen and present it to helper T lymphocytes.

2. **The answer is D.** Autoimmune responses can include the activities of antibody, as well as T cells. In many cases, however, the autoimmune response is a normal method for removing dead and dying tissues and would not be associated with pathology. When the mechanisms regulating normal autologous responses fail, the response can continue out of control, damaging critical tissues and causing autoimmune disease.

3. **The answer is C.** Antigen that cannot be processed and held by the MHC molecules is not able to stimulate CD4 lymphocytes and does not induce a secondary immune response.

4. **The answer is C.** Adjuvants, such as alum, bind the antigen molecules and maintain them in a concentrated particulate form. Macrophages are able to phagocytize particulate materials efficiently. Some adjuvants also function by inducing a local inflammatory response, thus recruiting inflammatory cells to the area of the immunization.

5. **The answer is D.** Mitogens are compounds that can stimulate mitosis in a variety of cell types. Some mitogens are plant lectins, such as concanavlin A and pokeweed mitogen. These materials bind and cross-link cell-surface carbohydrates, causing the target cell to undergo mitosis. Other mitogens perturb membrane structure and stimulate mitosis.

6. **The answer is A.** The set of cytokines elaborated in a superantigen response includes only those cytokines produced by macrophages and helper T cells.

7. **The answer is A.** Passive immunization provides the product of an immune response (i.e., antibody) to an individual. This procedure does not result in an active immune response, a secondary immune response, or immunologic memory.

8. **The answer is D.** Following a known exposure, it is important that immunologic protection be available more quickly than the organism can exert its pathology. Passive immunization provides immunity rapidly but needs to be followed by active immunization. Active immunization with either an attenuated vaccine or an appropriate protein vaccine representing the organism provides the long-term protection that is not available with passive immunization. However, there is a period of time during the generation of the active immune response when the individual is not protected.

9. **The answer is B.** Chemical modification of an autologous structure can induce an immune response. As a result of the immune effector mechanisms, the tissue containing the modified antigen can be damaged, exposing previously hidden or sequestered antigens. Any imbalance of the immune response, such as a cytokine imbalance or an abnormally intensive polyclonal response to an agent, has the potential of initiating autoimmunity.

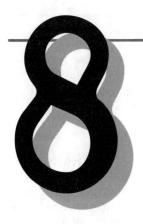

MAJOR HISTOCOMPATIBILITY COMPLEX

CHAPTER OUTLINE

INTRODUCTION OF CLINICAL CASE

Dr. Gonzales, a 56-year-old chemical engineer, was suffering from a progressive renal insufficiency and awaiting a kidney transplant. To identify the most suitable organ for the transplantation, the hospital laboratory tissue-typed Dr. Gonzales and identi-

Considering all of the possible allelic differences between two individuals, why is there an emphasis on matching the HLA-A, HLA-B, and HLA-C tissue types of the donor and recipient?

fied which specific human leukocyte antigens (HLA) he expressed. The laboratory results showed that Dr. Gonzales was tissue type HLA-A2, 23; HLA-B4, 12; and HLA-C7, 26.

ORGANIZATION OF THE MAJOR HISTOCOMPATIBILITY COMPLEX

The major histocompatibility complex (MHC) is a set of multiple genes, located on the short arm of human chromosome 6, that codes for proteins with significant growth and development functions. The genes for the class I and class II MHC molecules that we have been studying are found within the MHC. There are also genes that code for other proteins related to the immune response. For example, the genes for the C4 and C2 components of the classic complement pathway, for B factor found in the alternate complement pathway, and genes coding for critical cytokines such as tumor necrosis factor (TNF) are all found in the MHC. This third, more diverse set of genes is often referred to as coding for the class III MHC molecules. However, in this study of the basic principles of immunology, we concentrate only on the class I and class II molecules. The class III MHC molecules along with products of other genes found within the MHC have important activities in a variety of organ or development systems, and a study of their functions and expressions, although fascinating, is beyond the scope of this book.

Nomenclature

The term **antigen** is often used to discuss cell-surface structures. The terms differentiation antigens and class II MHC antigens refer to protein markers on the surfaces of some cell types and are used to distinguish those cells.

MHC nomenclature is complex. Historically, multiple names have been used to refer to both the MHC genes and their protein products. Moreover, these names vary when referring to the MHC of different species. The term MHC is generic and refers collectively to this gene complex in any species. Each species, however, has its unique name for the MHC. For example, the MHC complex of the human is referred to as the HLA complex. Although the name was derived from the gene products that were initially described on leukocytes, they are now known to be found on all nucleated cells. On the other hand, the MHC of the mouse, consisting of the same set of genes, is called the H2 complex and codes for H2 antigens.

Because the mouse has been the source of much information about the immune system, it is not surprising that mouse and human **nomenclature** for the MHC products are sometimes confused.

To complicate the issue of nomenclature further, the proteins associated with the MHC in each of the species are also referred to by different names. For example, the class I MHC molecules that are expressed on all nucleated human cells and present products of cellular synthesis to CD8 cytotoxic T lymphocytes are called HLA-A, HLA-B, and HLA-C antigens. On the other hand, class I MHC molecules performing an identical function in the mouse are called H-2K and H-2D antigens. There are similar differences in nomenclature of the class II MHC molecules. Human class II MHC proteins are referred to as HLA-DP, HLA-DQ, and HLA-DR proteins or antigens; mouse class II MHC genes are referred to as *H2-IA* and *H2-IE*, and the corresponding cell-surface proteins are the IA and IE antigens.

It is important to stress that, in both species, all the class I molecules are found on all nucleated cells, and they function in the presentation of products synthesized by the cell to CD8 cytotoxic T lymphocytes. The class II molecules, on the other hand, are found on a more restricted set of cells (antigen-presenting cells [APCs], B lymphocytes, activated T lymphocytes, and, at lower concentrations, on some other cell types) and present processed phagocytized antigen to the CD4 T lymphocytes.

The term *antigen* indicates how these markers were first discovered. In many cases, either polyclonal or monoclonal antisera generated by immunization with a unique cell or cell line was able to generate an antisera that reacted with a structure on the cell surface (an antigen). These antisera became extremely valuable tools to investigate both the structure and functions of the cells and cell-surface markers (antigens).

Sections of MHC Genes

Fig. 8-1 shows the general structure of the human MHC gene complex, illustrating the relative locations of the class I, II, and III genes. Clearly the structure of the gene complex is far more complicated than shown in Fig. 8-1. Not all of the genes are represented. Moreover, each of the individual genes within this structure has an organization of introns, exons, leader sequences, regulatory sequences, and untranslated sequences, like other eukaryotic genes. In addition, pseudogenes and other class I and II molecules are not illustrated and are not discussed.

Heterogeneity of MHC Genes

The characteristic of the MHC that kept Dr. Gonzales waiting for a kidney transplant was the polymorphism associated with the class I and II MHC gene products. Within the entire population, there are multiple alleles for each of the HLA class I (*HLA-A*, *HLA-B*, *HLA-C*) and class II (*HLA-DP*, *HLA-DQ*, *HLA-DR*) molecules, making this set of genes one of the most complex and heterogeneous gene systems known. Within the individual, however, there is far less diversity. As with the other eukaryotic genes, two copies of the chromosome are inherited, and both alleles for each of the class I and class II genes are expressed. Therefore, each cell capable of expressing the class I MHC molecules can display six different types: two alleles representing the *HLA-A* genes, two alleles representing the *HLA-B* genes, and two alleles representing the *HLA-C* genes are expressed. In the case of the *HLA-A* gene only, there are more than 50 different alleles present in the

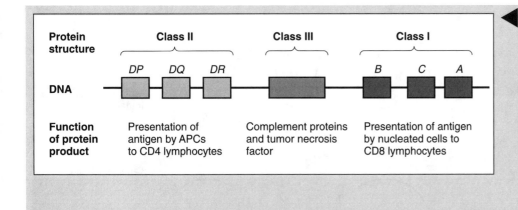

FIGURE 8-1
MHC Gene Regions in Human. This map lists only genes coding for proteins that are critical for the initiation of the immune response. There are three different class I MHC proteins expressed on nucleated cells, and the genes coding for these three different proteins are found in the HLA-A, HLA-B, and HLA-C regions of the MHC. There are also three different class II MHC proteins expressed on antigen-presenting cells, B cells, and activated T cells. The genes coding for these three different proteins are found in the HLA-DP, HLA-DQ, and HLA-DR regions of the MHC. A third class of MHC genes codes for some of the complement proteins and for tumor necrosis factor. There are genes for other class I and class II molecules, as well as other proteins, that are not identified in this figure.

population. Dr. Gonzales expresses only two of those *HLA-A* alleles. As Dr. Gonzales's immune system developed, it was "educated" to recognize his unique set of HLA-A molecules as one of the six antigen-presenting structures on all nucleated cells. A similar discussion can take place for each of the class I and class II MHC molecules. It is important to remember that Dr. Gonzales's immune system did not learn to recognize, as self, the other class I and class II alleles present in the population, which he does not possess.

It must be stressed that, although there are differences in the amino acid sequence and potential differences in the sets of processed peptides that can be displayed on the cell surface for each of the molecules in either the class I or the class II set, the functional properties (i.e., presenting antigen to either CD4 T lymphocytes in class II or CD8 T lymphocytes in class I) are identical for each individual molecule within the set.

*Allelic differences are commonly found when comparing proteins from different individuals. However, the **polymorphism** in the class I and class II MHC molecules is significantly greater than in any other gene system. What is the selective advantage for this high degree of polymorphism in the antigen-presentation machinery?*

RELATIONSHIP OF STRUCTURE TO FUNCTION

Class I MHC Molecules

Fig. 8-2 outlines the structure of a generic class I MHC molecule. This molecule consists of two polypeptide chains. One chain, the α chain, has a molecular weight of approximately 47,000 daltons. This molecule is a transmembrane protein in which the major portion of the molecule is found on the extracellular surface. The molecule has small cytoplasmic and transmembrane domains. The gene coding for the α chain is contained within the MHC, and all of the allelic heterogeneity of the class I molecule, discussed above, is contained within the α chain. The differences between the HLA-A, -B, and -C molecules also reside in the amino acid sequences of the α chain.

The second polypeptide chain in the class I MHC structure, having a molecular weight of 12,000 daltons, is a molecule called β_2-microglobulin. The amino acid sequence of β_2-microglobulin is consistent from one class I molecule to another. Moreover, β_2-microglobulin is also found in association with other cell-surface proteins that are not part of the cellular antigen-presentation mechanisms. The gene for β_2-microglobulin is not located within the MHC.

The three-dimensional structure of the class I molecule reflects its function in presenting antigen fragments to CD8 T lymphocytes. The α chain folds into three domains: α_1, α_2, and α_3. Both the α_3 domain and the β_2-microglobulin molecule have structures similar to immunoglobulin domains and are considered members of the immunoglobulin superfamily of genes. The α_1 and α_2 domains, however, display more of a globular structure and interact with each other to create the site that holds the

The RasMol home page at http://www.umass.edu/microbio/rasmol/ has a copy of the RasMol molecular viewer, which can be downloaded for a look at x-ray structures of the class I and class II MHC molecules.

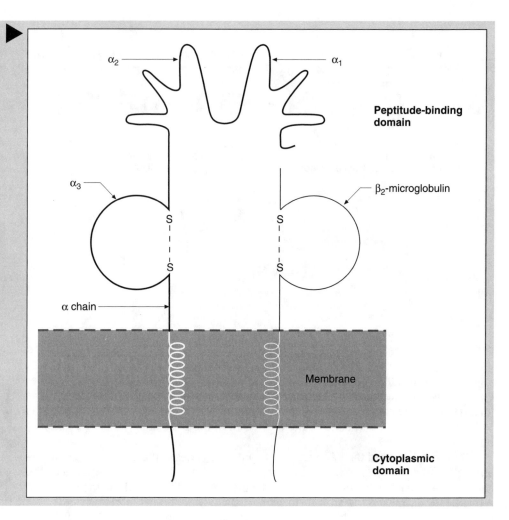

FIGURE 8-2 ▶

MHC Class I Molecule. *The molecule as it exists on the cell surface is composed of two polypeptide chains. The gene for the larger of the two chains, the α chain, is found in the MHC, while the smaller chain gene is located on a different chromosome. The α chain is a transmembrane protein that folds into a structure capable of binding and displaying processed peptide on the surface of all nucleated cells.*

processed peptide. Fig. 8-3 schematically illustrates the three-dimensional structure of the peptide-holding α_1 and α_2 domains. It is in the groove, illustrated in this figure, that the processed peptide antigen is displayed for the CD8 cytotoxic T lymphocyte.

Class II MHC Molecules

Fig. 8-4 schematically represents the structure of the class II MHC molecule. From a three-dimensional perspective, the molecule looks similar to the class I molecule discussed above, including the groove that holds the processed antigen. The class II molecule, however, has a different polypeptide configuration. In this structure, the α chain is approximately 34,000 daltons, and the β chain is only slightly smaller. Both polypeptide chains are transmembrane proteins. In contrast to the class I molecules, however, genes for the α and β of class II chains are both found in the MHC complex. This leads to a more complex gene structure for the *DP*, *DQ*, and *DR* segments of the MHC. Fig. 8-5 illustrates an expanded view of the DNA coding for the class II MHC molecules. The polymorphism of the class II MHC molecules is found in both the α and β chains.

In addition to the class II MHC α and β chains, a third polypeptide chain called the *invariant chain* is associated with the class II structure during synthesis and transport. The invariant chain is thought to play a role in protecting the peptide-binding site until an antigen peptide can be added to the site. The invariant chain is not associated with the MHC molecule that is expressed on the surface of APCs. Although the structure of the class II protein is remarkably similar to the class I protein, including the peptide-binding groove, the expression and function of the class II molecules are different. Class II molecules, as we have learned, present phagocytized antigen to CD4 T lymphocytes.

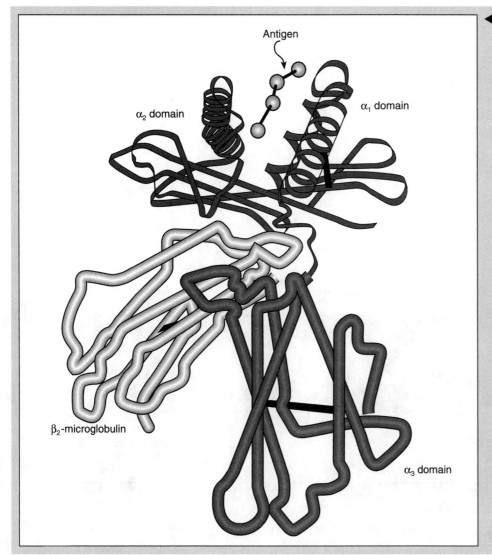

Antigen

α_2 domain

α_1 domain

β_2-microglobulin

α_3 domain

◀ FIGURE 8-3
Class I MHC Three-Dimensional Structure.
The β_2-microglobulin molecule and the α_3 domain of the heavy chain interact with each other to form a folding pattern much like the domain structure and interactions found in the immunoglobulin molecule. The α_1 and α_2 domains of the heavy chain possess more of a globular structure and fold to create an antigen-binding groove. Processed antigen peptide, as illustrated in the figure, fits into the groove and is displayed on the cell's surface.

FIGURE 8-4 ▶

Class II MHC Molecule. *The molecule as it exists on the cell surface is composed of two polypeptide chains, the α chain and the β chain. However, unlike the class I MHC molecule, both α and β chains are transmembrane proteins. The gene for both chains of the class II MHC structure are found in the MHC. The three-dimensional structure of the class II molecule is remarkably similar to the structure of the class I MHC molecule (see Fig. 8-3), including the presence of a peptide-binding groove.*

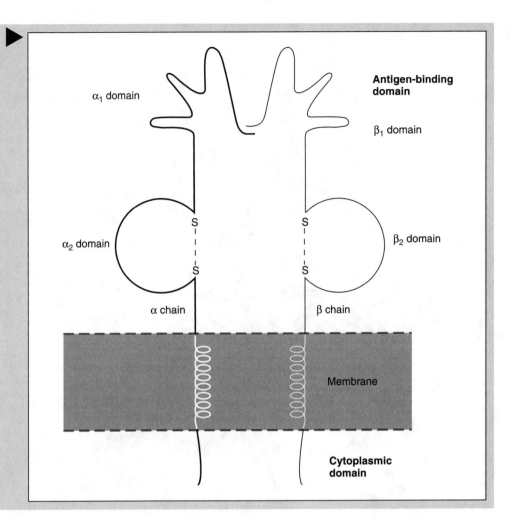

FIGURE 8-5 ▶

Class II MHC Gene. *The genes coding for the three different class I MHC α chains are located within the MHC. However the gene for β₂-microglobulin, an essential part of the class I structure, is located on a different chromosome. In contrast to the class I gene structure, genes for both the α and β chains of the class II MHC molecule are found in the MHC.*

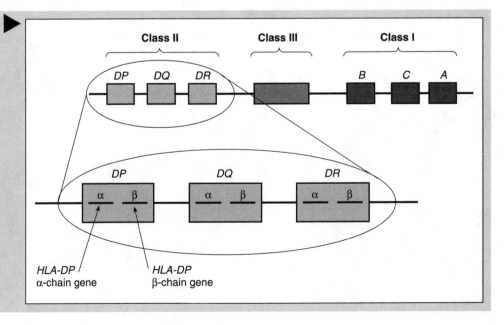

ANTIGEN-BINDING HETEROGENEITY OF CLASS I AND II MHC MOLECULES

One recurrent theme in this discussion of the MHC molecules has been the significant polymorphism exhibited by these proteins. For Dr. Gonzales, the polymorphism presents a major problem in his waiting for an acceptable donor organ. In a response to an antigen exposure for a single individual, the population polymorphism of the MHC proteins is not a major factor because an individual's immune system develops recognizing his or her own set of MHC molecules. For the individual to have a successful immune response to an infectious agent, his or her set of MHC molecules must successfully hold and present processed peptides. On the other hand, if the nature of the infecting antigen is such that it cannot be successfully presented by one of the individual's MHC molecules, that individual will not respond successfully to the infectious agent.

From the viewpoint of the population, however, the polymorphism of the MHC molecules has a definite selective advantage. Many of the polymorphic sites are located in or near the antigen-binding groove. This implies that the different alleles of any one of the MHC molecules may either hold and display the same antigen differently or may display an entirely different set of peptides. Consequently, because of the large degree of polymorphism in the population, there is a much greater possibility that some individuals will express MHC molecules capable of holding processed antigen from any infectious agent.

ANTIGEN PRESENTATION AND DISEASE

Because of the integral relationship between the MHC presentation of antigen and the eventual immune response, it is not unexpected that MHC type can play a critical role in an individual's response to disease. This relationship can take many forms in different situations.

Transplantation

Dr. Gonzales is an excellent example of the role that the MHC plays in health and disease. Should Dr. Gonzales receive a transplanted organ that displays foreign MHC allotypes, cells expressing the foreign molecules would continue to present antigen fragments of all synthesized proteins. However, Dr. Gonzales's immune system was "educated" to recognize his MHC types and has learned to tolerate self-proteins presented in the context of his own MHC. But now, the transplanted cell is presenting fragments of self-proteins in a totally different context, one that can and does stimulate an immune response to the self-antigen–foreign MHC allotype. Fig. 8-6 illustrates the differences between these two responses. In this case, the immune system is fooled into believing that all self-proteins presented on the foreign MHC molecules are foreign and to be eliminated. Consequently, a major cell-mediated immune response is directed toward cells expressing foreign MHC structures.

Tissue rejection because of differences between HLA-A, HLA-B, and HLA-C molecules and the corresponding HLA molecules expressed on the transplanted organ is primarily the result of CD8 cytotoxic T lymphocytes. Mismatch of the class II MHC molecules can also lead to rejection of the cells expressing the foreign class II molecules. For Dr. Gonzales, a mismatch of the class II molecules would have few consequences because of the limited tissue distribution of the class II MHC molecules. In this case, APCs within the foreign organ stimulate the host CD4 and, eventually, CD8 responses, resulting in the eventual elimination of the foreign APCs. Similarly, host APCs that invade the transplanted organ stimulate foreign CD4 cells that reside in the foreign organ to induce a response to the host. In this situation, there is a two-way mixed lymphocyte reaction (MLR) [Fig. 8-7]. The host's immune system responds to the graft, and the immunocompetent cells resident in the graft respond to the host. Because of the

MLR refers to the cellular immune reaction resulting from differences in class II MHC molecules. This reaction can take place either in vivo or in vitro. MLC refers to an MLR that takes place in an experimental tissue culture. The two terms MLR and MLC are often used interchangeably.

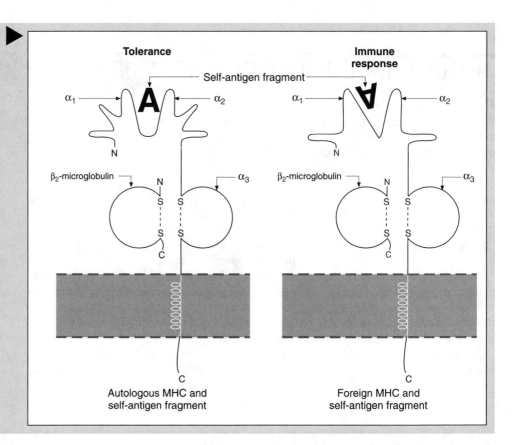

FIGURE 8-6 ▶

Differences between Autologous and Foreign MHC-presented Antigen. The manner in which the MHC molecules present antigen can have dramatically different effects on the eventual immune response. During development, the T-cell component of the immune system is "taught" to recognize what autologous molecules look like when presented on self-MHC molecules. The result of this education is tolerance or a carefully regulated immune response to autologous components. However, when the same autologous antigen fragment is presented in the context of a foreign MHC molecule, as in a transplanted tissue carrying a foreign MHC allotype, the antigen fragment can be bound and displayed in a conformation that is not recognized as self by the T cells. As a result, all antigens, both autologous and foreign, have the capacity to induce immune responses.

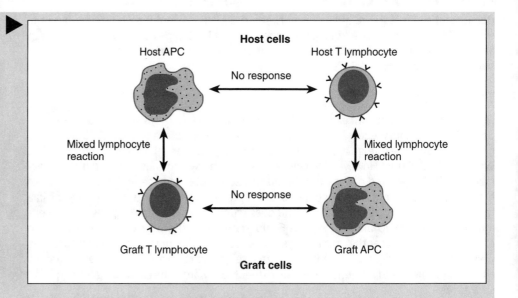

FIGURE 8-7 ▶

Mixed Lymphocyte Reaction. When immunocompetent cells from two individuals of different major MHC types are mixed, there is a mutual stimulation. This is a mixed lymphocyte reaction (MLR). During development, the T cells from each individual "learned" to distinguish between self- and foreign antigens in the context of the common MHC type. However, the T cells of the host have not learned to recognize self-antigen in the MHC type of the grafted tissue, and the T cells resident in the grafted tissue have not learned to recognize self-antigen in the MHC type of the host. The reaction that is produced by mixing leukocytes from individuals with different MHC types stimulates proliferation of both host and graft T cells and leads to the mutual destruction of both sets of cells. APC = antigen-presenting cell.

overwhelming size of the host's immune system, the outcome of the two reactions is the elimination of the immunoresponsive cells that were resident in the grafted tissue. This entire reaction can be reproduced in the laboratory by culturing together leukocytes from two different individuals, and the magnitude of the responses from the resulting mixed lymphocyte culture (MLC) can be quantitated and used for investigating immune responsiveness.

For Dr. Gonzales, the removal of the graft's immune system is of little functional significance unless there is collateral damage to the other functional cells of the transplanted organ. However, in a case where an active immune system is transplanted into an immunosuppressed patient, the outcome can be very different. In such a scenario, the host would have no immune system to counterattack the immunocompetent cells of the graft, and the graft would reject the host. This is graft-versus-host (GVH) disease. In contrast to the problem of class II incompatibility in Dr. Gonzales's kidney transplant, if there were a class I incompatibility on the transplanted tissue, Dr. Gonzales's immune system would respond immunologically to all cells in the organ, eventually leading to a major episode of tissue rejection.

Associations between HLA and Disease

Associations have been discovered between certain diseases and different HLA allotypes. These associations have been found for both the class I and class II molecules. The rationale for the HLA associations is not always clearly defined. However, it is relatively easy to imagine how presenting one unique antigen in a different HLA context may give rise to very different results. For example, in one HLA type, the HLA–antigen complex may resemble an important self-structure and alter the normal immune regulation to that structure, whereas in another HLA type, presentation of the same antigen has no similarity to the normal structure. In the former case, infection or exposure to the offending antigen could result in an autoimmune response; in the second case, the offending antigen would be eliminated by the immune system without consequence. One of the best examples of the role of HLA in disease comes from the studies of type I diabetes mellitus. In this case, when the unknown antigen is presented by an HLA molecule that contains a small amino acid residue (e.g., serine or alanine) at a specific location in the antigen-binding site, there is a higher probability for the individual to develop an autoimmune response to the β cells of the pancreas. However, should that residue be replaced in a different HLA type with a large amino acid (e.g., aspartic acid), then there is resistance to the disease.

RESOLUTION OF CLINICAL CASE

Dr. Gonzales eventually received an organ transplant that was matched at all of the *HLA-A*, *HLA-B*, and *HLA-C* alleles, except one. As part of his transplant follow-up therapy, he was put on a regimen of immunosuppressant medications to prevent rejection of the transplanted organ. During the course of his continued recovery, the dosage of his anti-inflammatory medications was reduced. He experienced several episodes in which his CD8 cytotoxic T lymphocytes began to mount an immune response to the transplanted organ. For each episode, it was necessary to increase the anti-inflammatory therapy to prevent tissue rejection.

In each of the rejection episodes, the MHC molecules on the cells of the transplanted tissue expressed fragments of normal proteins. However, these molecules are displayed in the context of the altered MHC-binding pocket and therefore are presented to the immune system in an unexpected conformation. In this situation, even protein fragments produced by the transplanted tissue, which are sequentially identical to Dr. Gonzales's own proteins, are regarded by the immune system as foreign when displayed in the context of foreign MHC. Dr. Gonzales's physician faces an ongoing challenge to administer anti-inflammatory agents that can control episodes of tissue rejection while maintaining sufficient immune system activity, so that other essential immunologic functions continue.

REVIEW QUESTIONS

Directions: For each of the following questions, choose the **one best** answer.

1. Which of the following sets of MHC molecules can be detected on the surface of a fibroblast isolated from a kidney?
    (A) HLA-A, HLA-B, and HLA-C
    (B) HLA-DP, HLA-DQ, and HLA-DR
    (C) Molecules in both sets (HLA-A, HLA-B, HLA-C; HLA-DP, HLA-DQ, HLA-DR) would be detected.
    (D) Molecules representing only one member in set HLA-A, HLA-B, HLA-C would be detected but not all three.
    (E) Molecules representing only one member in set HLA-DP, HLA-DQ, HLA-DR would be detected but not all three.

2. Which of the following sets of MHC molecules can be detected on the surface of a macrophage (Langerhans' cell) isolated from the skin?
    (A) HLA-A, HLA-B, and HLA-C
    (B) HLA-DP, HLA-DQ, and HLA-DR
    (C) Molecules in both sets (HLA-A, HLA-B, HLA-C; HLA-DP, HLA-DQ, HLA-DR) would be detected.
    (D) Molecules representing only one member in set HLA-A, HLA-B, HLA-C would be detected but not all three.
    (E) Molecules representing only one member in set HLA-DP, HLA-DQ, HLA-DR would be detected but not all three.

3. Unlike antibody molecules, the MHC molecules do not exhibit allelic exclusion. Which of the following statements is a direct consequence of this difference?
    (A) A somatic cell expresses only one of the HLA-A, HLA-B, or HLA-C proteins.
    (B) A somatic cell expresses all three of the class I MHC molecules.
    (C) A somatic cell expresses two different types of the HLA-A molecule.
    (D) Since antibody is secreted and MHC molecules are found on the cell surface, allelic exclusion is of no relevance.

4. Which of the following statements about the class I and class II MHC molecules is correct?
    (A) Both the class I and the class II MHC molecules have an identical cellular distribution.
    (B) A single cell may express either a class I or a class II MHC molecule, but not both.
    (C) In spite of the fact that the molecules are composed of different polypeptide chains, the final three-dimensional structure of both class I and class II molecules is remarkably similar.
    (D) Because the processing pathway for both molecules is different, the final three-dimensional structure of the two classes of molecules must be significantly different.

5. A child's tissue type is HLA-A2,23; HLA-B5,13; and HLA-C4,7. The mother's tissue type is HLA-A4,23; HLA-B5,17; and HLA-C2,7. Which of the following is the father's tissue type?

    (A) HLA-A4,23; HLA-B5,13; and HLA-C2,7

    (B) HLA-A2,13; HLA-B13,27; and HLA-C4,14

    (C) HLA-A6,23; HLA-B5,12; and HLA-C4,6

    (D) HLA-A2,13; HLA-B5,12; and HLA-C2,7

6. Which of the following statements is correct concerning the function of a foreign MHC molecule on a transplanted tissue?

    (A) Because the transplanted MHC molecule is foreign, it cannot be expressed on the transplanted tissue.

    (B) Although the foreign MHC molecule is expressed, it cannot function to present antigen to the host's immune system.

    (C) The foreign MHC molecule on a transplanted tissue can be expressed and present antigen, but the host's immune system does not respond because of the allotype differences.

    (D) The foreign MHC molecule on a transplanted tissue can be expressed and present antigen, and the host's immune system can respond to the MHC-presented antigen.

7. An individual who is missing both B-cell and T-cell immunity (severe combined immunodeficiency syndrome) received a transplant of bone marrow stem cells in an attempt to reconstitute his immune system. The cell donor was of a different MHC allotype, and the grafted bone marrow cells were contaminated with mature lymphocytes. Which of the following is the most likely outcome of this transplant?

    (A) The transplant should be successful because the host cannot reject the donor cells.

    (B) The transplant would not be successful because the donor cells will reject the host tissue.

    (C) Although the donor stem cells would survive, they are not able to repopulate the host immune system because the developing lymphocytes cannot recognize the HLA molecules of the host.

    (D) As a result of the HLA difference, the host will reject the donor cells.

8. Antisera that reacts with β_2-microglobulin can be used as a tool to identify which of the following molecules?

    (A) All class I MHC molecules

    (B) All class II MHC molecules

    (C) Only the HLA-A molecules

    (D) Only the HLA-DR molecules

9. Which of the following is a correct statement about the MHC gene complex?

    (A) In addition to containing genes that code for the class I and class II MHC molecules, the complex contains genes that code for complement components, cytokines, and other proteins not directly related to the immune system.

    (B) The gene complex contains genes for the MHC proteins, the antibody molecules, and the T-cell receptor.

    (C) The gene complex only contains genes related to the immune system.

    (D) Only the genes coding for the MHC proteins are found in the complex.

ANSWERS AND EXPLANATIONS

1. **The answer is A.** All nucleated cells express both alleles of the class I MHC molecules. Consequently, on a fibroblast isolated from a kidney, there would be examples of six different class I MHC molecules. The examples include two allelic types of HLA-A, two allelic types of HLA-B, and two allelic types of HLA-C.

2. **The answer is C.** Antigen-presenting cells (APCs) are nucleated cells and express both alleles of the class I MHC molecules. In addition, macrophages also express the class II MHC molecules so that they can present antigen to CD4 T lymphocytes. As a result, the APCs express six different types of class I MHC molecules and six different types of class II MHC molecules: two allelic types of HLA-DP, two allelic types of HLA-DQ, and two allelic types of HLA-DR.

3. **The answer is C.** The antibody molecule is somewhat unique in that only one allele of the gene is expressed. This is biologically important, because it prevents a single B cell from making two totally different antibodies when selected by a single antigen. The MHC molecules, on the other hand, do not exhibit allelic exclusion. This is biologically important, because it can increase the number of different antigen-binding structures on a cell surface. Consequently, there are molecules representing both alleles of the *HLA-A*, *HLA-B*, and *HLA-C* genes.

4. **The answer is C.** In spite of the fact that the polypeptide composition is different, the class I and class II MHC molecules exhibit a remarkably similar three-dimensional structure. The molecules, however, have different cellular distributions and present antigen to different cell types. Antigen-presenting cells express both classes of the MHC molecule.

5. **The answer is B.** The child inherited the HLA-A23, HLA-B5, and HLA-C7 allotypes from the mother. All remaining class I allotypes in the child, HLA-A2, HLA-B13, and HLA-C4, must be inherited from the father.

6. **The answer is D.** The MHC system is active in all functional, nucleated vertebrate cells. This system is continually processing and presenting either synthesized protein (class I MHC) or phagocytized antigen (class II MHC). The foreign MHC can then present antigen fragments to the host's immune system. The difference in bound antigen conformation gives rise to the host's immune response to that antigen.

7. **The answer is B.** In this situation the host cannot mount an immune response and reject the foreign cells. However, donor cells containing mature lymphocytes have the potential to recognize differences in the host cells and initiate an immune response to the host. This is an example of graft-versus-host disease.

8. **The answer is A.** All class I MHC molecules are associated with β_2-microglobulin. In addition to its association with the class I MHC molecules involved in antigen presentation, β_2-microglobulin is an integral component of the structure of other cell-surface proteins that have a structure similar to the class I MHC molecules but have functions outside of the immune system.

9. **The answer is A.** Although immunology studies tend to focus on the class I and class II genes in the MHC complex, the complex includes a very complicated set of genes coding for proteins active in several phases of the immune response as well as proteins not directly related to the immune response. This complex does not, however, include the genes coding for either the antibody molecule or the T-cell receptor.

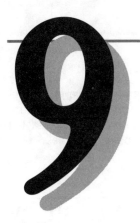

STRUCTURE OF ANTIBODY AND LYMPHOCYTE ANTIGEN RECEPTORS

CHAPTER OUTLINE

INTRODUCTION OF CLINICAL CASE

Mrs. Jones, a 56-year-old woman with chronic fatigue, consulted her physician. During the past year, she contracted more infections than usual and recently began experiencing generalized body aches with prominent skeletal pains. Because of the gradual onset of her symptoms, she could not relate her problems to any single event or time. Physical examination was normal except for elevated blood pressure. Laboratory testing identified a normochromic and normocytic anemia, with slightly elevated serum calcium level. A significantly elevated serum protein concentration that exhibited a markedly low serum A:G ratio was also found. In addition, the patient exhibited proteinurea. To further investigate the bone pain, her physician ordered a series of x-ray studies, and the results showed numerous patches of low density that looked like holes punched out of the bone.

An electrophoresis study performed on Mrs. Jones's serum (Fig. 9-1) disclosed a

FIGURE 9-1 ▶

Serum Electrophoresis Study. A sample of Mrs. Jones's serum was placed in a matrix that was connected to a power source. The proteins in the serum separated, based on their intrinsic charge. The positively charged proteins migrated to the negative electrode, and the negatively charged molecules migrated to the positive electrode. This procedure separates serum into albumin, α-globulin, β-globulin, and γ-globulin zones. Mrs. Jones's serum (solid line) shows an abnormally high level of γ-globulin with a prominent spike of protein. In addition, there is a slight decrease in the albumin fraction. Normal serum is indicated by the dashed line.

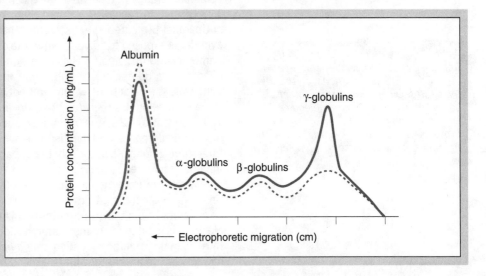

sharp spike of protein in the γ-globulin region. The protein in the urine, however, was not identical to the serum protein when characterized by either molecular weight or electrophoretic mobility. Nevertheless, both the serum protein and the urine protein reacted with antibodies that were capable of binding human immunoglobulin molecules.

STRUCTURE OF A GENERIC ANTIBODY

Monoclonal Gammopathy
The elevated level of γ-globulin results from a single type of antibody molecule from a single clone of cells.
Polyclonal Gammopathy
The elevated level of γ-globulin results from many different types of antibody molecules from several different clones of cells.

The data in the above clinical case are consistent with a monoclonal gammopathy, in which an elevated level of immunoglobulin (myeloma protein) from a single clone of antibody-producing cells is found in the blood. The structure of this monoclonal protein is identical to the immunoglobulin molecule that was previously discussed (Fig. 9-2). Myeloma proteins were, in fact, the source of the material that eventually led to the elucidation of antibody structure. The molecule consists of two identical heavy chains with molecular weights of approximately 50,000 daltons each and two identical light chains of approximately 25,000 daltons each.

FIGURE 9-2
Structure of a Generic Myeloma Protein.
The structure of a generic myeloma protein consists of two identical light chains and two identical heavy chains. In addition, the domain folding structure of the molecule and the disulfide bonding pattern are indicated in this figure. —SS— = disulfide bond.

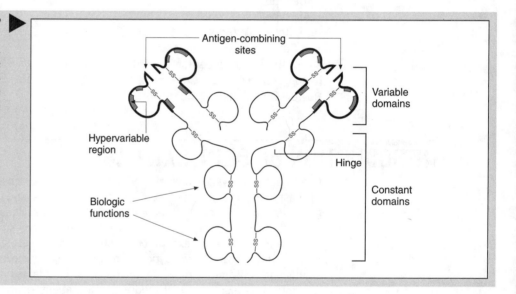

A large family of proteins, including the immunoglobulin molecule, the T-cell receptor for antigen, portions of the HLA molecules, along with several other cell-surface and cell-adhesion molecules, employ the **immunoglobulin folding motif**. Proteins without known relationship to the immune system also use this type of folding pattern.

When analyzed, the three-dimensional structure of the myeloma protein shows a common folding pattern in both the light and heavy chains. This pattern defines a 12,000-dalton repeating domain (Fig. 9-3). Each of these protein domains forms an antiparallel β-pleated sheet structure that takes the form of a cylinder. One side of the cylinder is exposed to solvent, while the other face of the cylinder interacts with another immunoglobulin domain. The three-dimensional representation of the molecule is derived from a composite of both light and heavy chains (Fig. 9-4). In addition to the noncovalent interactions within and between domains holding the molecule in its final three-dimensional structure, there are intradomain and interdomain disulfide bonds. This composite of a stable immunoglobulin folding pattern, interactions between immunoglobulin domains, and the disulfide bonding pattern provide the molecule with a stable three-dimensional structure that is capable of functioning in the harsh environment of inflammatory sites.

When the immunoglobulin molecule (see Fig. 9-4) is treated for short periods of time with proteolytic enzymes, the amino-terminal light- and heavy-chain domains can be separated from the carboxyl-terminal heavy-chain domains (Fig. 9-5). The proteolytic cleavage is located in an unstructured section of the heavy chain between the second and third domains, which is called the *hinge*. The hinge allows a significant amount of mobility of the amino-terminal domains relative to the carboxyl domains and facilitates

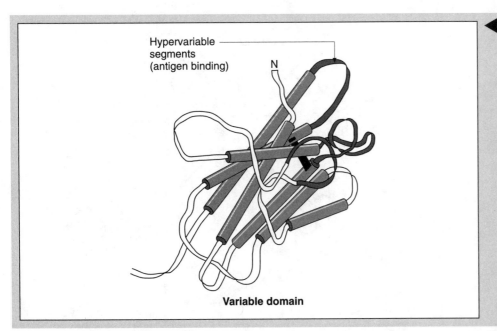

FIGURE 9-3

Three-Dimensional Structure of a Single Immunoglobulin Domain. *The polypeptide chain folds into a barrel-like structure, with the polypeptide chain tracing an antiparallel, β-pleated-sheet pathway around the surface of the barrel. The intradomain disulfide bond crosses through the center of the structure. A similar folding pattern is observed in both the variable and constant domains. The folding pattern allows the amino acid sequences that make up the antigen-binding site to be arranged into a single contiguous surface. This structure is called the immunoglobulin fold and is a folding pattern found in several proteins.*

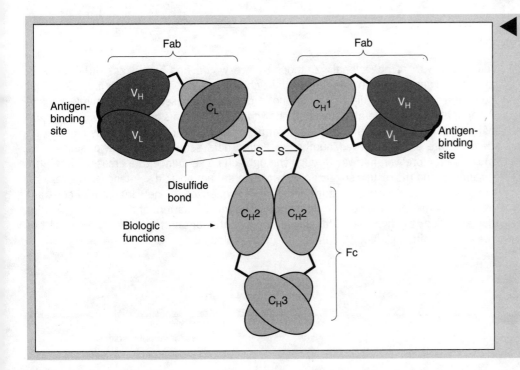

FIGURE 9-4

Three-Dimensional Structure for the Intact Immunoglobulin. *In this structure, one face of each domain interacts with solvent, while the other face is involved in binding to either a light- or heavy-chain domain. Both the light and the heavy chains contribute surfaces that create the antigen-binding site. Note the relatively unstructured region between the Fab and Fc portions of the molecule. In the figure, V refers to variable domains on either the light (V_L) or heavy (V_H) chains. The constant domains are indicated by C_L and C_H for the light and heavy chains, respectively. The heavy chains consist of multiple constant domains.*

antibody binding to sterically hindered antigens. The amino-terminal proteolytic fragment, called the *Fab fragment*, contains both light and heavy chains and is capable of binding antigen. When the two Fab fragments are connected by a disulfide bond, the resulting 100-dalton molecule is the $F(ab')_2$ fragment. Both Fab portions of the molecule are capable of binding antigen. The carboxyl-terminal fragments, which crystallize relatively easily, comprise the *Fc fragment*.

The nomenclature derived from the studies above describes different immunoglobulin locations. These names are used extensively when discussing the biologic function of antibody because many functional properties of the molecules are uniquely associated with either the Fab or Fc locations.

The studies of amino acid sequencing identify additional locations within the immunoglobulin's three-dimensional structure. If we compare the light-chain amino acid sequence of Mrs. Jones's myeloma protein to a light-chain sequence from another

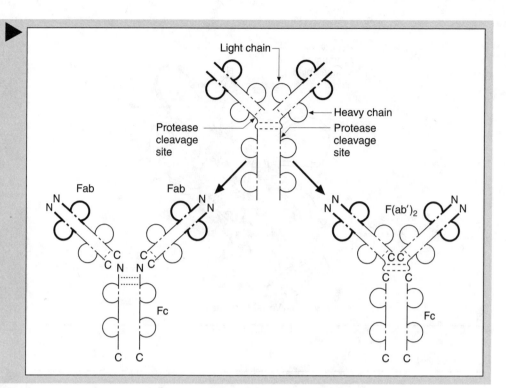

individual with a monoclonal gammopathy, we would find significant differences in amino acid sequence between the two light-chain proteins. Continuing this analysis and comparing Mrs. Jones's light-chain amino acid sequence to sequences from hundreds of other light chains, generates the chart shown in Fig. 9-6. This chart identifies segments of hypervariability along the light-chain sequence as well as regions in the sequence that demonstrate a more limited number of amino acid sequences in the population of molecules. Moreover, halfway through the light-chain sequence, the areas of variability disappear, and the results suggest only two different amino acid sequences. The regions of variable and relatively constant amino acid sequences define variable and constant domains of the immunoglobulin light chain. The folding pattern of the immunoglobulin domain brings the hypervariable regions into a contiguous surface that becomes part of the antigen-binding site in the intact antibody molecule.

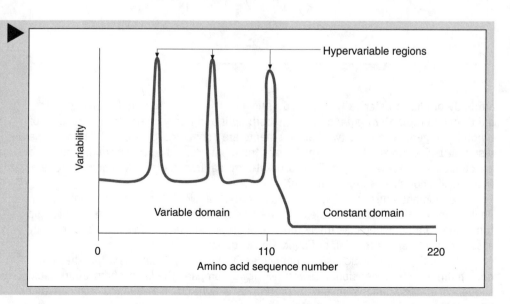

The constant domains identify two different types of light chains called κ and λ chains. Both κ and λ chains exhibit an amino-terminal variable domain with hypervariable segments, followed in the sequence by the κ or λ constant domains.

A similar pattern appears in the heavy chain. In this case, the constant domains identify five different types of heavy chains. The heavy-chain constant domains define the μ, δ, γ, ε, and α heavy chains, which are part of the immunoglobulin M (IgM), IgD, IgG, IgE, and IgA molecules, respectively. The light and heavy chains are associated and align the hypervariable regions, creating an intact antigen-binding surface.

At the RasMol home page, http://www.umass.edu/microbio/rasmol/, the student can view x-ray structures of the immunoglobulin molecule in the different presentation formats.

ANTIGENIC DETERMINANTS ON IMMUNOGLOBULINS

The amino acid sequencing studies provide evidence for two different types of light chains and five different types of antibody heavy chains. Similar results were obtained when purified human monoclonal antibodies and antibody fragments were used to immunize animals. In this case, the animal responds to the foreign (human) protein by making antisera, which specifically bind to surface structures that are unique to the monoclonal protein that was the immunogen. A collection of antisera, each reactive with different monoclonal human antibodies, provides useful reagents for investigating similarities and differences between different human antibody molecules. This immunization approach identified three different types of immunoglobulin antigenic structures: isotypes, idiotypes, and allotypes.

Isotype

The immunoglobulin heavy chains (μ, δ, γ, ε, α) define, in part, the immunoglobulin isotype. The term *isotype* also refers to the type of light chain (κ, λ) that is associated with the heavy chain. A complete isotype description of an intact IgG molecule containing two λ light chains and two γ heavy chains would be $\lambda_2\gamma_2$. Similarly, an isotype description of an IgM molecule containing κ light chains would be $\kappa_2\mu_2$. It should be stressed that, in any normal immunoglobulin molecule, both heavy chains are identical and both light chains are identical. Moreover, either κ or λ light chains can be associated with any of the heavy-chain isotypes. There are different subtypes of the heavy-chain isotypes that generally represent differences in either the immunoglobulin hinge or disulfide-bond pattern. Different heavy-chain subtypes of the IgG molecule are called the γ1, γ2, γ3, or γ4 chain, whereas different heavy-chain subtypes of the IgM molecule are called the μ1 or μ2 chain.

All isotypes bind antigen. The antibody couples this antigen-binding function to different biologic functions. Each of the antibody isotypes is responsible for different sets of biologic functions (see Part 1). Table 9-1 outlines the chemical, physical, and biologic properties of the five immunoglobulin isotypes.

Isotype
This term refers to differences in immunoglobulin classes. IgM, IgD, IgG, IgE, and IgA represent the different immunoglobulin classes or isotypes. In all normal individuals, molecules can be identified from each of the five heavy-chain isotypes and both of the light-chain isotypes.

Idiotype

A second type of antigenic structure on the immunoglobulin molecule is the idiotype. The three-dimensional structure of the immunoglobulin molecule folds such that the hypervariable regions of the immunoglobulin are brought into a common surface, creating the unique antigen-binding site. The idiotype of an immunoglobulin can be most simply thought of as this antigen-binding surface. Therefore, the idiotype of a molecule represents the unique characteristics associated with the antigen-binding surface. During the course of an immune response, the antibody isotype, or class, changes from IgM of the primary response to IgG, IgE, or IgA of the secondary response. However, both the IgM primary antibody and the IgG, IgE, or IgA secondary antibody bind to the same antigen and share a common idiotypic structure.

The nature and immunology of the idiotypes is a fascinating area of advanced study. The idiotypic structures are of critical importance to the immunoregulatory mechanisms. Because of the extremely low concentration of each unique idiotype prior to antigen exposure, immunologic tolerance to the idiotype is not generated. Therefore, we generate

Idiotype
This term refers to differences between antibody molecules that identify characteristics of the antigen-binding site. As the secondary immune response matures, affinity of the antibody for the antigen increases. During affinity maturation, there are changes in the nature of the idiotype that reflect the change in antigen binding.

TABLE 9-1 ▶
Properties of the Immunoglobulin Isotypes

Property	IgM	IgD	IgG	IgE	IgA
Percent of total serum immunoglobulin concentration	9	0.2	75	0.004	15
Serum concentration (mg/dL)	120	3	1000	0.05	200
Sedimentation coefficient	19s	7s	7s	8s	8s, 10s, 11s
Molecular weight	900k	180k	150k	190k	170k, 360k, 400k
Structure	Monomer (B-cell receptor) and pentamer	Monomer	Monomer	Monomer	Monomer and dimer
Heavy-chain type	μ	δ	γ	ε	α
Complement fixation	+	−	+	−	−
Placental transport	−	−	+	−	−
Mediation of allergic responses	−	−	−	+	−
Major secretory antibody	−	−	−	−	+
Opsonization	−	−	+	−	−
B-cell receptor for antigen	+	?	−	−	−

an autoantibody response to the idiotypic portions of our own antibody molecules. The autoantibody is called anti-idiotypic antibody.

Allotype

The third type of antigenic site on immunoglobulins is the allotypic marker. Whereas the isotypic and idiotypic markers are unique to the immunoglobulin molecule, with analogous structures on the T-cell receptor (TCR), allotypic markers are a common feature of all proteins. The allotypic markers are inherited substitutions of a few different amino acid residues in the background of the antibody isotype. In the population, the light chains and each of the heavy-chain isotypes have a set of associated allotypic markers. For example, the markers associated with the γ heavy chain are called Gm markers (Gm1, Gm2, . . .), and the allotypic markers associated with the κ light chain are called Km markers (Km1, Km2, . . .). Similar nomenclature is applied to the other immunoglobulin polypeptide chains. Whereas the population contains all of the allotypic markers, each individual within the population expresses only the allotypic markers that he or she inherited.

Because of the unique nature of the different immunoglobulin markers, different immunization protocols can be used to produce anti-isotype, antiallotype, and anti-idiotype antisera. Immunizing across species identifies major differences between the immunoglobulin polypeptide chains and gives rise to primarily anti-isotype antisera. Immunizing between individuals of the same species gives rise to primarily antiallotype antisera, and returning high concentrations of a purified antibody into the individual who produced the molecule results in an anti-idiotype response.

LYMPHOCYTE ANTIGEN RECEPTORS

Both T and B lymphocytes express antigen-specific receptors that are members of the immunoglobulin gene superfamily of molecules. In the case of the B lymphocyte, the antigen receptor is a monomeric form of the IgM molecule. In the case of the T lymphocyte, the antigen receptor is a molecule with significant structural homology to the antibody molecule, consisting of both variable and constant domains. On the cell surface, both B-cell and T-cell antigen receptors must be coupled to other membrane proteins that help transmit signals to the interior of the cell that an antigen-binding event has taken place.

B-Cell Antigen Receptor

This cell-surface form of the IgM molecule is only slightly different from the secreted 19s pentameric IgM. In the cell-surface molecule, the carboxyl-terminal amino acids that allow the molecule to polymerize into a pentamer have been replaced by a membrane-spanning domain. For the information that the B cell has bound antigen to reach the interior of the lymphocyte, the B cell's membrane-bound IgM molecule must be associated with signal transduction mechanisms (Fig. 9-7). The protein kinases are associated with that function. If any of the components of this B-cell antigen receptor are missing, the modified B cell will function aberrantly.

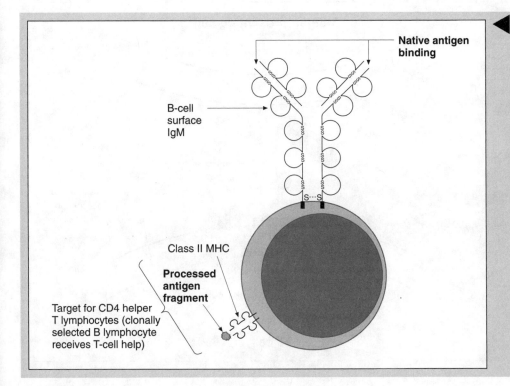

◀ FIGURE 9-7

B-Cell Antigen Receptor. The B lymphocyte binds antigen via its cell-surface IgM or via IgM and IgD molecules. The antigen is internalized, along with the antibody receptor, and processed. Fragments of the processed antigen are presented in association with the B cell's class II MHC molecules, and this structure serves as a recognition site to allow CD4 helper T cells, which have been stimulated by the same antigen, specifically to deliver the required cytokines to the selected B lymphocyte.

A second type of antigen receptor expressed on the B-lymphocyte surface is the class II major histocompatibility complex (MHC) molecule. Antigen that has been specifically bound by the lymphocyte IgM receptor is internalized, processed, and presented on the B cell's class II molecules. This serves as an antigen structure that the activated CD4 helper T lymphocytes can use to deliver specifically the cytokines that are necessary for eventual proliferation, isotype switching, and further differentiation of the selected B lymphocyte. In summary, activation of a B lymphocyte, leading to a secondary response, requires two events: (1) specific antigen binding by the cell-surface IgM antigen receptor and (2) antigen presentation to an activated antigen-specific CD4 helper T cell.

T-Cell Antigen Receptor

The TCR is not a classic immunoglobulin molecule, although it has several similarities and is a member of the immunoglobulin family. The α and β chains of the TCR are composed of immunoglobulin-like variable and constant domains. The variable domains of the TCR carry the unique specificity that allows the T lymphocyte to bind the class II MHC molecule and processed antigen complex.

The T lymphocyte requires multiple interactions between the TCR and antigen-presenting structures on the antigen-presenting cell (APC) surface (Fig. 9-8). These interactions are necessary to stimulate the cell. The CD3 molecules are associated with the TCR α and β chains and are necessary for signal transduction. In addition, intercellular adhesion molecules (ICAMs) and differentiation antigens also exhibit binding interactions during the clonal selection of T lymphocytes. There are also binding reactions that are unique to each type of presenting cell. If the presenting cell is displaying the class II MHC molecule, the CD4 molecule found on the helper T cell binds to the class II MHC molecule. If the presenting cell is displaying the class I MHC molecule (i.e., a target for a CD8 cytotoxic T cell), the CD8 molecule found on the cytotoxic T cell binds to the class I MHC molecule. Collectively, this set of interactions creates surfaces inside both cells that can activate the protein kinases of the signal transduction systems. Failure to make these interactions successfully results in alterations of the final immune response and even tolerance to the antigen.

FIGURE 9-8 ▶

T-Lymphocyte Antigen Receptor. The T-cell receptor (TCR) for antigen is a heterodimer consisting of α and β polypeptide chains, having a structure very much like the Fab fragment of the immunoglobulin molecule. This is the portion of the TCR that binds to the MHC antigen fragment on the antigen-presenting cell (APC). A set of proteins necessary for signal transduction called CD3 is associated with the TCR. To achieve a productive immune response, several other interactions between accessory molecules on the T cell and the cell presenting the antigen must take place. In addition, there are interactions unique to each type of presenting cell. Most notable are the interactions between CD4 and the class II MHC molecule of the APC as well as those between the CD8 and the class I MHC molecule, which is the target of the cytotoxic T lymphocyte..

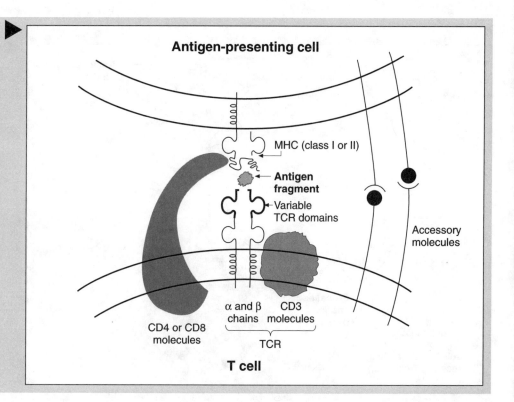

RESOLUTION OF CLINICAL CASE

Mrs. Jones's overproduction of a unique monoclonal antibody resulted from a plasma cell tumor. In this plasma cell dyscrasia, multiple myeloma, the metastatic events happen in a single cell that is making antibody of a unique idiotype. Clones of that initial cell proliferate uncontrollably in the bone marrow and other tissues, and each continually produces its specific antibody product. When a plasma cell produces antibody, there is coordination in the amount of light and heavy chain produced. However, in some myelomas, one of the chains is overproduced. In Mrs. Jones's case, there is overproduction of the light chain, resulting in the production of intact antibody and an excess of light chain. The excess light chain folds into the proper three-dimensional conformation for an immunoglobulin domain. However, since there are no heavy chains with which to associate, the excess light chains often aggregate with each other and are secreted from the myeloma cell. Because of their smaller size and higher concentrations, these light-chain monomers and dimers, called Bence-Jones proteins, are found in the urine.

In Mrs. Jones's case, the damage to the bones, indicated in the x-ray, resulted from the clones of the myeloma cell that became established in the bone marrow. The myeloma cells displaced normal bone and interfered with the functions of the bone marrow. The patient's anemia resulted from the myeloma cells displacing normal erythropoiesis. It would also be expected that the other bone marrow–derived blood cell populations would be adversely affected, which may be the cause of her increased incidence of infections. Mrs. Jones's slightly increased blood pressure is due, in part, to the myeloma protein that has increased plasma protein concentration and subsequently plasma viscosity.

Mrs. Jones was referred to an oncologist, who initiated antineoplastic therapy in an attempt to reduce and eventually eliminate her myeloma cells.

REVIEW QUESTIONS

Directions: For each of the following questions, choose the **one best** answer.

1. Which of the following is the most accurate description of the isotype of an IgG molecule that contains κ light chains?

    (A) $\kappa\mu$

    (B) $\kappa_2\mu_2$

    (C) $\kappa_2\delta_2$

    (D) $\kappa_2\gamma_2$

    (E) $\kappa_2\varepsilon_2$

2. Which of the following is a repeating unit of molecular structure found in all members of the immunoglobulin gene superfamily of molecules?

    (A) The light chain

    (B) The heavy chain

    (C) The complex between light and heavy chains

    (D) The immunoglobulin fold, as represented in an immunoglobulin domain

    (E) The globular Fab and Fc fragments, connected by an unstructured hinge

3. The portions of the immunoglobulin structure that come together to create the unique antigen-binding site include which of the following segments?

    (A) The constant segments of light and heavy chains

    (B) The hypervariable segments of light and heavy chains

    (C) The hypervariable segments of the light chain

    (D) The hypervariable segments of the heavy chain

    (E) The constant segments of the heavy chain with variable segments of the heavy chain

4. Antigen-binding activity of the immunoglobulin molecule is found in which of the following locations?

    (A) The hinge

    (B) The Fab fragment

    (C) The Fc fragment

    (D) The carboxyl-terminal domain

    (E) The groove where the two Fab fragments connect to the hinge

5. An IgG antibody molecule was discovered that was able to inhibit competitively the binding of an IgM antibody to its antigen. Upon further testing, it was discovered that the IgG molecule did not bind to the antigen but did bind to the IgM molecule. Which of the following antibodies best describes the IgG antibody?

    (A) Anti-isotype antibody

    (B) Anti-idiotype antibody

    (C) Antiallotype antibody

    (D) Anti-Fab antibody

    (E) Anti-Fc antibody

Note. Abbreviations used in the questions: IgG = immunoglobulin G; Fab = amino-terminal fragment; Fc = carboxyl-terminal fragment; TCR = T-cell receptor; MHC = major histocompatibility complex; IgM = immunoglobulin M;

6. Injecting a purified IgG-λ myeloma protein into a rabbit primarily produces antisera that react with which of the following determinants?

   (A) Idiotypic determinants

   (B) Allotypic determinants

   (C) Isotypic determinants on the heavy chain

   (D) Isotypic determinants on the light chain

   (E) Isotypic determinants on both the heavy and light chains

7. Transfusion of plasma from one individual to another, unrelated individual primarily will produce antisera that react with which of the following determinants?

   (A) Allotypic determinants

   (B) Isotypic determinants on the heavy chain

   (C) Isotypic determinants on the light chain

   (D) Isotypic determinants on both the heavy and light chains

8. Antigen is found on B lymphocytes associated with which of the following molecules?

   (A) Only the B-cell IgM antigen receptor

   (B) Only the B-cell class II MHC molecules

   (C) Both the cell-surface IgM molecule and the class II MHC molecules

   (D) Neither the cell-surface IgM molecule nor the class II MHC molecules

9. Antibody production is stimulated by clonal selection of an appropriate B lymphocyte. Which of the following statements correctly describes the binding activity of the antibody?

   (A) The antibody binds to the class II MHC antigen fragment expressed on the surface of the B cell that responded to the antigen.

   (B) The antibody does not bind to the class II MHC antigen fragment expressed on the surface of the B cell that responded to the antigen.

   (C) The antibody binds to the class II MHC antigen fragment expressed on a macrophage presenting the same antigen.

   (D) The antibody binds to the TCR of a T cell that responds to the same antigen.

   (E) The antibody is an anti-idiotype antibody.

10. Antisera to which of the following cell-surface molecules is able to detect all T lymphocytes?

   (A) Anti-CD4

   (B) Anti-CD8

   (C) Anti-CD3

   (D) Anti-Fab

   (E) Anti-IgM

ANSWERS AND EXPLANATIONS

1. **The answer is D.** The isotype is a description of the polypeptide chains that comprise an immunoglobulin molecule. For an IgG molecule that contains κ light chains, the intact molecule would contain two identical γ heavy chains and two identical κ light chains.

2. **The answer is D.** The immunoglobulin fold, as represented in the structure of a domain, is a repeated protein-folding motif. This folding pattern is found in the TCR, MHC molecules, cell-adhesion molecules, and other molecules without known connections to the immune system. Both the heavy and light chains of the immunoglobulin express this folding pattern in the structures of their domains. Molecules like the MHC proteins express this immunoglobulin folding pattern in only some of their domains and have different folding patterns in other sections of the molecule.

3. **The answer is B.** The antigen-binding site of the antibody molecule or the TCR is a composite surface, generated by the hypervariable segments of both the light and heavy chains of the antibody or the α and β chains of the TCR. The constant segments of the immunoglobulin domains are structural, in that they help maintain an appropriate structure to either hold the hypervariable domains in a contiguous surface or maintain the sections of the antibody molecule that mediate the biologic functions in an active conformation.

4. **The answer is B.** Antigen binding occurs near the amino-terminal portion of the light and heavy chains. Although the hinge may play an important function in allowing antibody to bind hindered or sterically inaccessible antigens, it does not participate directly in the interactions with antigen. The Fc fragments and carboxyl domains of the molecule also contain functional sites. However, these sites are related to the biologic functions of the molecule, not to antigen binding.

5. **The answer is B.** Antibodies that block antigen binding react in or near the antigen-binding surface (i.e., the idiotype). This is best described as an anti-idiotype antibody. The antigen-binding surface of many immunoglobulins is rather large and represents approximately 5%–10% of the antibody's surface. If the antigen is small, portions of the binding surface may not be occupied by the antigen and anti-idiotype antibody, so the unoccupied portions of the surface do not block antigen binding.

6. **The answer is E.** When immunizing across species, all determinants on both the heavy and light chains can induce immune responses. In addition, idiotypic determinants and allotypic determinants induce responses. However, these are minor in comparison to the number of isotypic structures.

7. **The answer is A.** Immunizations between different individuals generate immune responses to allotypic sites. This is found not only for the immunoglobulin molecules but also for the allotypes found in all proteins. To produce an anti-idiotypic response would require isolating and purifying the antibody product of a single clone of B lymphocytes and immunizing the individual who produced that antibody with their own antibody. For example, Mrs. Jones, in the clinical case, would be expected to produce an anti-idiotype response to her myeloma protein.

8. **The answer is C.** During the stimulation of a B lymphocyte, antigen is initially bound to the cell-surface immunoglobulin receptor. The antigen-receptor complex is internalized, processed, and presented in association with the B-cell class II MHC molecules.

9. **The answer is B.** The surface immunoglobulin of the B lymphocyte recognized the three-dimensional structure of the antigen. Once this molecule is processed by proteolytic fragmentation, the three-dimensional character of the antigen as recognized by the antibody is lost. Consequently, the antibody response to an antigen will not react with either the class II MHC–antigen complex or the TCR that reacts with the identical antigen.

10. **The answer is C.** Antisera to the variable regions of the TCR will be antigen dependent. Since all T lymphocytes possess the CD3 molecules that are a necessary part of the signal transduction mechanisms, CD3 is used as a marker for all T lymphocytes. The CD4 molecules are only found on helper T cells, and the CD8 molecules are only found on cytotoxic T lymphocytes.

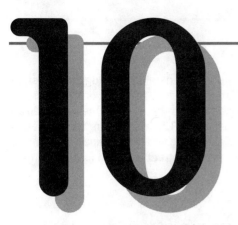

GENERATION OF ANTIBODY AND T-CELL RECEPTOR DIVERSITY

CHAPTER OUTLINE

INTRODUCTION OF CLINICAL CASE

John Franklin is a 46-year-old civil engineer who was rushed to the emergency room with a high fever, dehydration, and hemorrhaging from his mouth and nose. He had been working on a construction project in a remote, South American location when he became ill, and he was rushed home for treatment. Serologic analysis failed to identify an antibody response to any known viral or bacterial agent. Moreover, blood bacterial and viral cultures were not successful in identifying the causative agent. Mr. Franklin was started on a course of antibiotic treatment, which produced no measurable improvement in his condition.

ORGANIZATION OF THE IMMUNOGLOBULIN GENE

In the clinical case, Mr. Franklin has been infected with an unidentified agent. Antibiotic therapy was unsuccessful, and there are no reagents available to provide him some measure of protection by passive immunization. In this situation, Mr. Franklin must rely on the ability of his humoral and cellular immune systems to generate a sufficient antigen-binding diversity to insure a response to this new agent.

One of the unique characteristics of the immune response is the specificity with which the antibody or the T cell reacts with the antigen. The hypervariable nature of the combining site for antigen suggests that a cassette model is employed for the construction of the immunoglobulin. In this model, hypervariable antigen-binding segments are inserted into an immunoglobulin or T-cell receptor (TCR) framework that holds the hypervariable regions in the proper configuration to react with antigen. When a new antigen is encountered, antigen-binding diversity is generated by plugging different cassettes (hypervariable sequences) into the static framework. In reality, antigen-binding diversity is generated at the DNA level in the absence of antigen, when the bone marrow stem cell differentiates into either B or T lymphocytes. The mechanism for generating antigen-binding diversity is remarkably similar to the cassette model and involves randomly selecting different minifragments of genes to construct the gene for the eventual antibody or TCR molecule.

Light-Chain Gene

Fig. 10-1 outlines a simplified structure for the germline configuration of an immunoglobulin light-chain gene. This complex shows multiple V (variable) gene segments and a limited number of J (joining) gene segments, which eventually, through DNA rearrangements and RNA splicings, produce a messenger RNA (mRNA) that directs light-chain synthesis. There are approximately 250 V segments, 4 J segments, and 1 gene segment representing the constant domain (either κ or λ). The gene coding for each of the light chains (κ or λ) is essentially identical in the configuration of the V, J, and constant gene segments.

FIGURE 10-1 ▶

Germline Configuration of the Immunoglobulin Light-Chain Gene. The gene consists of hundreds of variable (V) segments and at least four available joining (J) segments for each constant (κ or λ) gene. The exact number of gene segments varies among species and also varies between the κ and λ light-chain gene systems. Diversity is generated by selecting any one of the V segments and ligating it to any one of the J segments.

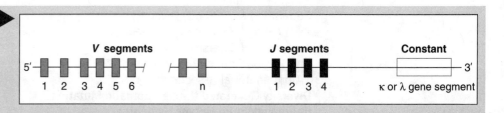

Upon receiving the appropriate growth and differentiation signal, the stem cell becomes committed to either the B- or T-cell lineage. Similar processes happen in both T- and B-cell development. In this discussion we will follow B-cell differentiation. An integral part of that commitment step is the rearrangement of the immunoglobulin light-chain gene, which randomly selects one of the V segments and ligates it to any one of the J segments (Fig. 10-2). Each time a stem cell starts down this differentiation pathway, there is a similar rearrangement of V and J segments. If the specific V–J combination changes, the resulting antibody will exhibit different antigen-binding properties.

Fig. 10-1 and Fig. 10-2 are oversimplifications of the immunoglobulin gene. There are signal sequences both prior to and following each of the V and J sequences. These signal sequences help achieve a productive alignment of the V and J segments. In addition, there are protein leader sequences in front of each of the V segments. These sequences are common to all secreted proteins, and they help direct the newly synthesized proteins to the proper cellular compartment. The resulting rearranged DNA segment is transcribed into RNA, and with eventual RNA splicing and processing, an mRNA is produced that codes for the light chain of the immunoglobulin.

Heavy-Chain Gene

The mRNA from which the heavy chain of the immunoglobulin is transcribed is constructed from a similar set of DNA rearrangements and RNA splicings. The heavy-chain gene, however, is more complicated than the light-chain gene in two important respects. First, the heavy-chain gene has an additional set of gene fragments, the D segments, which can increase diversity of the final heavy-chain variable region. The second major difference is in the organization of the gene fragments that code for the constant portions of the molecule. There is one set of V, D, and J gene fragments for all five of the heavy-chain isotypes. The organization of the variable segments of the immunoglobulin heavy-

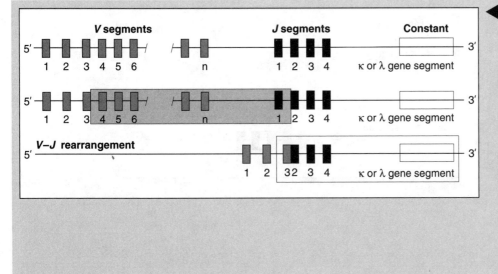

FIGURE 10-2

Generation of Diversity by V–J Rearrangement. During the differentiation of the bone marrow stem cell into a B lymphocyte, the germline structure of the light-chain DNA is rearranged. This rearrangement involves ligating one of the variable (V) segments to one of the joining (J) segments. In this figure, V segment number 3 is ligated to J segment number 2. The nuclear material between these two gene segments (shaded box) is removed to produce the rearranged V–J light-chain gene that is observed in the mature B lymphocyte. The segment of the gene that is the template for RNA transcription is outlined by the unshaded box. The RNA is processed to remove the unused J segments and DNA sequences that are unnecessary for protein synthesis. In the process, the rearranged V–J segments are ligated directly to the 5' of the light-chain constant gene segment.

chain gene is outlined in Fig. 10-3. Genes that code for the constant domains of all five heavy chains—μ, δ, γ, ϵ, and α isotypes—sequentially follow the V, D, and J gene segments (Fig. 10-4). In the unstimulated B cell the rearranged VDJ segment is adjacent to the gene segment coding for the μ-chain of IgM. Upon receiving T-cell help, a secondary immune response, the rearranged VDJ segment is moved such that it is adjacent to either the gamma segment (IgG response), the epsilon segment (IgE response) or the alpha segment (IgA response).

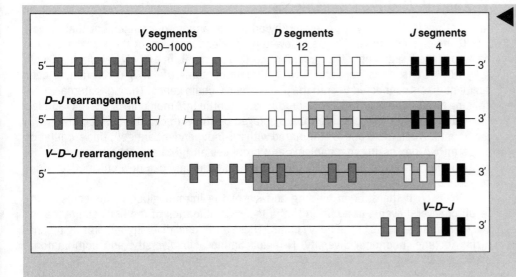

FIGURE 10-3

Germline Configuration of the Immunoglobulin Variable Domain. Like the light-chain gene, the heavy-chain variable domain consists of from hundreds to thousands of variable (V) segments and at least four available joining (J) segments. In addition, there is a set of 12 diversity-generating D segments. The process of DNA rearrangement of these gene fragments happens during the initial differentiation and development of the B cell. Initially, there is a D–J rearrangement. During this rearrangement, the D and J segments between the ligated pair (shaded box) are lost. Following the initial D–J rearrangement, a V gene segment is randomly chosen to ligate the newly rearranged D–J segments. Again, the intervening V and D segments (shaded box) are lost. In the mature B lymphocyte, the V–D–J segments have been rearranged to produce the structure in the last line of the figure.

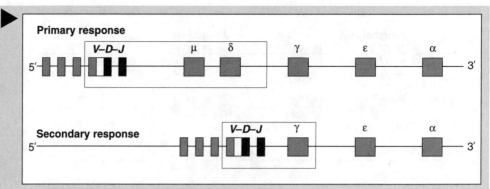

FIGURE 10-4 ▶

Immunoglobulin Gene as Rearranged in the Primary and Secondary Immune Response. In the mature B lymphocyte, the rearranged V–D–J segments are closely associated with the gene segments coding for μ and δ heavy chains. The RNA transcript that is produced is indicated by the dotted line. *Messenger RNA (mRNA) is produced from this initial transcript by processing and splicing events. By altering the RNA splicing at the 3' end of the μ gene, either membrane or secreted forms of the IgM molecule can be produced. Once the B lymphocyte has received T-cell help and the information to direct the switching of isotypes, there is a second rearrangement of the heavy-chain DNA. In this case, the rearranged V–D–J gene segments that were initially next to the 5' end of the μ heavy-chain gene are moved to the 5' end of the γ heavy-chain gene with the resulting loss of the μ and δ gene segments. The unshaded box around the secondary response gene indicates the DNA that codes for the RNA transcript of the IgG heavy-chain gene.*

GENERATION OF ANTIBODY DIVERSITY

V–J and V–D–J Rearrangements

Antigen-binding diversity is generated by an initial random rearrangement that selects one *D* and one *J* segment. This is followed by a selection of one of the *V* segments and ligation of the *V* segment to the newly formed *D–J* segment. In a newly developing B cell, the mRNA transcribed from this DNA template contains the *V–D–J* rearranged gene segment that is connected to both the μ and δ heavy-chain genes. Through alternate RNA splicing events, the resulting B cell produces either the IgM molecule or the IgM and IgD molecules. These molecules are then displayed on the extracellular surface of the cell membrane. When the B cell is stimulated with a T-independent antigen, this stimulation alters mRNA-processing mechanisms and produces an IgM heavy chain that does not contain the membrane-binding domain. As a result, the IgM can now polymerize and is secreted.

Diversity in the antigen-binding surface of the immunoglobulin molecule is the result of several events in addition to the *V–J* recombination of the light chain and the *V–D–J* rearrangements of the heavy chain. These additional diversity-generating mechanisms include junctional diversity, N-region amino acid diversity, and combinatorial association.

Junctional Diversity

When the *V* and *J* or the *V, D,* and *J* gene segments ligate, there is flexibility in the ligation reaction. To keep the proper sequence of the resulting protein, the triplet structure of the DNA code must be maintained. There are several ways to maintain the triplet code. For example, when ligating *V* and *J* segments, all three nucleotides for the amino acid code can be derived from one of the partners and none derived from the other. Alternatively, two nucleotides could be derived from one partner and one nucleotide derived from the other partner. All of these permutations may lead to a different amino acid in the final protein and to differences in the hypervariable segments.

N-Region Amino Acid Diversity

For the gene rearrangements discussed above to occur, several ligations of gene fragments must take place between V, D, and J segments. The ligation reactions can result in the loss or addition of nucleotides that are not coded for by the germline DNA. This diversity-generating mechanism, the noncoded or N-region amino acids, further increases the variability of an antibody's combining site for antigen.

Combinatorial Association

It must be remembered that the light chains and the heavy chains rearrange independently and randomly. Any one rearrangement of a heavy chain is free to associate with any rearrangement of the light chain. Therefore, while the heavy chain in one developing B cell may associate with the light chain of one specific sequence, a second B cell, one that by chance makes an identical heavy chain, creates a different antigen-binding specificity if that heavy chain associates with a light chain having a different V–J rearrangement. It must be emphasized that all of the diversity-generating mechanisms discussed above take place during the development of the B cell and in the absence of antigen. Table 10-1 summarizes how these events work together to generate a vast diversity in antigen-binding potential.

◀ **TABLE 10-1**
Mechanisms Generating Antibody Diversity

	Heavy Chain	*Light Chain (λ)*
V–J and V–D–J rearrangements		
V segments	250–1000	250 (2 κ chain)
J segments	4	4 (3 κ chain)
D segments	12–13	0
Number of combinations	$\sim 10^4$	$\sim 10^3$
Junctional diversity	+	+
N-region diversity	+	Low
Combinatorial association of light and heavy chains	$\sim 10^7$	
Estimated total diversity considering all mechanisms	$\sim 10^9$–10^{11}	

Note. The numbers in the table are estimates derived from the mouse immunoglobulin gene. The corresponding human gene appears to be larger.

DIVERSITY GENERATED THROUGH SOMATIC MUTATION

In addition to antigen-binding diversity that is generated during the differentiation and development of the bone marrow stem cell, additional binding diversity can be generated during the maturation of an ongoing immune response. It is currently thought that this diversity is the result of a somatic mutation that occurs during DNA replication and cell proliferation. During clonal expansion, the vast majority of the progeny of the selected B cell express identical idiotypes, which represent the idiotype of the original B lymphocyte. However, if a somatic mutation increases the affinity of the antibody, then, in the presence of additional antigen, the cell that expresses the new high-affinity idiotype is selectively stimulated. This continued clonal selection results, in part, in the affinity maturation observed during the shift from a primary to secondary response.

IMMUNOGLOBULIN ISOTYPE SWITCHING

The antibody-combining site for antigen is randomly generated prior to antigen exposure. However, during an antibody response to antigen, the isotype of the antibody produced switches as the primary response matures into a secondary response. This process of changing antibody isotypes, while maintaining the unique antigen-binding specificity (i.e., idiotype), again involves rearranging the immunoglobulin gene. On the heavy chain, the combined *V–D–J* segment, which was initially in proximity to the μ and δ heavy-chain gene segments, must be moved next to a heavy-chain gene fragment representing one of the other antibody isotypes. Regulatory factors supplied by the T lymphocyte direct the nature and type of isotype switch. In this process (see Fig. 10-4), the *V–D–J* gene segment is religated to a location proximal to a gene representing either the γ, ε, or α heavy-chain isotype. The nuclear material that originally coded for the IgM and IgD molecules appears to be irreversibly lost in this isotype switch. In Fig. 10-4, the initial isotype switch was from IgM to an IgG isotype. Presumably, under the influence of additional T-cell factors, the antibody-producing cell can undergo another gene rearrangement and switch to making either IgE or IgA. Because the information (gene) for making the preswitch antibody isotype is lost, a cell making an IgE or IgA antibody is prevented from reverting to making an IgG molecule.

ORGANIZATION OF TCR GENES

The TCR for antigen is also a member of the immunoglobulin gene superfamily of molecules and, like the antibody molecule, consists of variable and constant domains. Hypervariable sequences within the variable domain are also present. There are five different isotypes that are associated with the antibody molecules, but there are only two types of TCRs. The most common form has α and β polypeptide chains, while the other, less abundant form is composed of different polypeptide chains called γ and δ chains. The gene structure for the TCR is more complicated than that for the antibody molecule. In the human, the δ gene segments are located within the α-chain gene region of chromosome 14. The β and γ chains are separate gene regions on chromosome 7, which is very much analogous to the immunoglobulin genes. In spite of the increased complexity of the gene structure, the mechanism of generating diversity (i.e., *V–D–J* and *V–J* recombination) is identical to that of the antibody molecule. For the TCR, it appears that the α and γ chains are analogous to the immunoglobulin light chain because the gene complex consists of *V*, *J*, and a constant gene segment. In contrast, the δ and β chains are similar to the heavy chain because diversity is generated from *V*, *D*, and *J* gene segments.

RESOLUTION OF CLINICAL CASE

Although Mr. Franklin was extremely ill as a result of the unknown agent, he was eventually able to recover. The antibiotics that he was given did not appear to alter the course of disease, except to decrease the possibility that he might contract a secondary infection.

While he was working on the construction project in South America, Mr. Franklin was infected with a newly discovered virus. Although he had no prior exposure to the organism and was never immunized to the agent, his immune system was capable of generating sufficient diversity to react with this new virus. Since, in Mr. Franklin's case, pre-existing immunity to the specific virus did not exist, the virus was given a significant period to establish the infection. During this period, virus concentration increased until a specific clone of antigen-reactive cells was selected. The specificity of either the T-cell receptor or B-cell receptor was generated prior to viral exposure by *V–J* and *V–D–J* rearrangements, N-region diversity, and by different combinatorial associations between light and heavy chains. As this specific clone of the antigen-reactive cells proliferated in response to viral stimulation, somatic mutation mechanisms allowed the antigen receptors to alter their combining site for antigen. This process has the potential to either increase or decrease the affinity for antigen. If the affinity for antigen increases, Mr. Franklin will be able to respond to lower concentrations of antigen. In addition, because of the increased number of antigen-specific cells, Mr. Franklin will be able to respond to the same virus more rapidly upon second exposure, and he will experience less severe symptoms.

REVIEW QUESTIONS

Directions: For each of the following questions, choose the **one best** answer.

1. Which of the following is a correct statement about the origin of antibody diversity?

    (A) Antigen exposure is necessary prior to the generation of the antibody's combining site for antigen.

    (B) Because B-cell and T-cell antigens are different, different mechanisms are employed to generate antibody and TCR diversity.

    (C) Somatic mutation of the antibody-combining site for antigen plays no role in the affinity maturation of a B-cell response.

    (D) Antigen-binding specificity is developed early in the B-lymphocyte differentiation process and in the absence of antigen.

2. The term combinatorial association refers to which of the following diversity-generating mechanisms?

    (A) Combining light-chain *V* and *J* gene segments

    (B) Combining heavy-chain *D* and *J* gene segments

    (C) Combining heavy-chain *V* and *D–J* gene segments

    (D) Combining light- and heavy-chain proteins to produce the intact antibody

3. When light-chain and heavy-chain gene segments are ligated during the rearrangement process, the ligase must couple the two partners while maintaining the triplet code. This can be achieved by selecting three bases from one partner and none from the other or by selecting two bases from one partner and one base from the other partner. This is an example of which of the following diversity-generating mechanisms?

    (A) Gene-segment rearrangements

    (B) Junctional diversity

    (C) N-region diversity

    (D) Combinatorial association

4. The amino acid sequence of a myeloma protein contained five additional amino acid residues that could not be accounted for by the germline configuration of the gene. This diversity-generating mechanism is best described as which of the following?

    (A) Gene-segment rearrangements

    (B) Junctional diversity

    (C) N-region diversity

    (D) Combinatorial association

5. An immune response will switch from the IgM isotype to the IgG isotype if

    (A) the time since exposure is long enough for switching to take place

    (B) the antigen is the type that gives rise to IgG responses

    (C) T-cell help to direct the switch is available

    (D) the route by which the host is exposed positively affects switching

Note. Abbreviations used in the questions: TCR = T-cell receptor; IgM = immunoglobulin M; MHC = major histocompatibility complex; IgA = immunoglobulin A; IgG = immunoglobulin G.

6. Following the first exposure to an antigen, the host produced an IgM response, which was followed by an IgA response. Later in life, following a second exposure to the identical antigen, the response was primarily of the IgG isotype. Which of the following best explains the response to the second exposure?

   (A) Isotype switching of the memory cells from an IgA response to the IgG response

   (B) Rearrangement of the heavy-chain gene in the memory cell, such that the V–D–J segment is placed next to the gene for the γ heavy chain

   (C) Because the γ and ε are lost during the isotype switch to the IgA response, the response following second exposure cannot possibly happen as described.

   (D) The IgG response is most probably the result of a new immune response, in which IgM was the antibody found early in the response.

7. Which of the following statements concerning the TCR gene is correct?

   (A) In order to save space in the genome, the TCR generates diversity by using the immunoglobulin V, D, and J gene segments.

   (B) Antibody and TCR use different mechanisms to generate antigen-binding diversity.

   (C) Because the TCR only needs to recognize class I or class II MHC, it does not require the extent of diversity that is found in the immunoglobulin molecule.

   (D) Although the diversity-generating mechanisms are identical, there is no association between the immunoglobulin gene system and the TCR gene system.

8. Which of the following correctly describes the differences between the genes for the variable domain of the immunoglobulin heavy and light chains?

   (A) Both gene systems use the same library of V segments, however, each gene system has its own unique set of J segments.

   (B) Both gene systems use the same library of V and J gene segments. The heavy chain is different because it has its own unique set of D genes.

   (C) The gene systems for the heavy and light chains are separate and independent.

   (D) Rearrangements in the heavy chain allow only certain, specific rearrangements in the light chain.

ANSWERS AND EXPLANATIONS

1. **The answer is D.** One of the key characteristics of the immune system is that antigen-binding specificity is developed prior to exposure to the antigen, and the antigen selects the appropriate B cell or T cell. The diversity-generating mechanisms of both B cells and T cells are identical despite the difference in antigen characteristics.

2. **The answer is D.** Choices (A), (B), and (C) are examples of gene rearrangements. Combinatorial association is a method of generating antigen-binding diversity, in which any single heavy chain is free to associate with any light chain to create an intact antigen-binding site.

3. **The answer is B.** There are multiple approaches to maintaining the DNA triplet code during a ligation process. As a result of the multiple ligation methods, the amino acid code at the junctions of the V and J segments or the V, D, and J segments vary significantly. This is the meaning of junctional diversity.

4. **The answer is C.** N-region diversity identifies sections of the amino acid chain where there is no corresponding gene segment in the DNA. Apparently, the repair and ligation methods of DNA can randomly fill in gaps or even excise nucleotide sequences where gene segments are rearranged. There appear to be different mechanisms for the rearrangement of light and heavy chains because N-region diversity is not as prevalent in light chains, when examined, as it is in heavy chains.

5. **The answer is C.** The T lymphocyte is absolutely essential in the progression from the primary to the secondary response. The T cell provides the information necessary to direct specifically the type of isotype switch.

6. **The answer is D.** During the process of isotype switching, gene segments coding for heavy-chain constant regions are lost. Consequently, a cell making an IgA response cannot revert to making an IgG response. In the scenario described in the question, antigen most likely stimulated an entirely new immune response by selecting a mature IgM-bearing B lymphocyte instead of an IgA memory cell. The difference in the response could be the result of a different route of antigen exposure or of the relatively short immunologic memory of IgA responses.

7. **The answer is D.** The diversity-generating mechanisms of the TCR are similar to those of the B cells. These two independent systems do not share genes or gene fragments.

8. **The answer is C.** Like the differences between the immunoglobulin gene system and the TCR gene system, the genes coding for the heavy chain and the light chain are independent, and rearrangements made by one gene do not affect the rearrangements of the other gene.

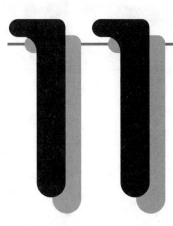

IMMUNOGLOBULIN E REACTIONS

INTRODUCTION OF CLINICAL CASE

Jane Henley is a 4-year-old child who, while playing outside, received an insect bite on her forearm. Moments after receiving the bite, the area around the injury began swelling rapidly and turned red. The injury was edematous with a large area of erythema around the site of the bite. Because of the rapid reaction, Jane was rushed to the urgent care facility. Jane's mother had never seen such a rapid and dramatic reaction, and she assured the physician that Jane had never received an insect bite of this type. Before the day was over the reaction to the bite began to subside. However, the next day Jane complained that the wound itched. Her mother noted that the swelling had returned, only now, the involved area was much larger, and the nature of the swelling was different. Instead of being edematous, as it had been immediately following the bite, the area of swelling was indurated.

> **Wheal and Flare**
> In cutaneous anaphylactic reactions, there is a soft (edematous) swelling called a **wheal**. The wheal is surrounded by an area of erythema called a **flare**.

BIOLOGIC ROLE OF IgE REACTIONS

The "inoculation" that Jane received as a result of the insect bite initiated a cascade of events that took place over the course of several days. When evaluated carefully, at least two different phases of Jane's reaction can be identified (Fig. 11-1). The first phase was immediate, requiring seconds to minutes, and edematous. The second phase of the response took longer (1 day) to develop and resulted in a larger swelling that was firm and not edematous.

Both the speed and the biphasic nature of the response are characteristic of an immunoglobulin E (IgE)–mediated reaction. Table 11-1 identifies some examples of IgE reactions. All of these reactions share the characteristics that were exhibited in Jane's response to the insect bite, and a similar chart could be generated for each example given

FIGURE 11-1 ▶

Time Course of an IgE Inflammatory Response. *This chart follows the time course of Jane's response to the insect·bite by measuring the diameter of the swollen tissue. The two phases of IgE reactions are clearly evident. There is an initial rapid edematous swelling, followed by a slower accumulation of lymphocytes, monocytes, and eosinophils, which gives the swelling a more indurated consistency.*

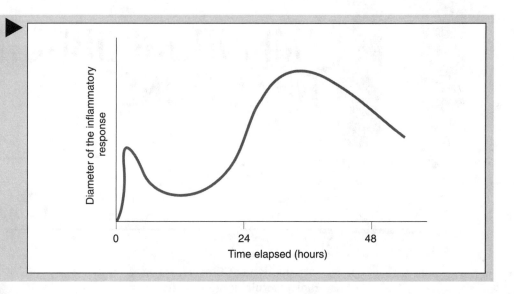

Individuals who are under a physician's care are statistically at greater risk of experiencing major anaphylactic reactions because treatment protocols often involve the administration of reactive drugs (e.g., penicillin) and biologic reagents.

in Table 11-1. This list is extensive and indicates the prevalence of IgE reactions throughout the world. IgE reactions are a major health concern and, when the reactions are systemic, can result in significant morbidity and possibly death. One, often mistaken interpretation of IgE reactions is that they are abnormal and should not take place. This is incorrect. IgE reactions are a normal and necessary immunologic protective mechanism. Only a hyperresponse or a chronic response has associated adverse and continuing pathology.

TABLE 11-1 ▶

Examples of IgE Reactions

Atopic Disease	Anaphylactic Disease
Allergic asthma	Systemic anaphylaxis
Allergic rhinitis	Urticaria-angioedema
Atopic dermatitis	
Allergic gastroenteropathy	

*Both the **IgE system** and the **complement system** produce a rapid inflammation that brings inflammatory cells to the site of the insult.*

*The IgE system also functions in immune protection against **helminths**. Antibody to the helminth can direct eosinophils to the target parasite. The major basic protein of the eosinophil granule is toxic to multiple cell types, including the helminth.*

One function of the IgE system is rapidly to inform the cells and factors of the immune system that a previously encountered antigen has been reintroduced. This activity can be likened to the duties of a sentry, who sounds a warning in the event of trouble. In Jane's case, foreign antigens (insect proteins) were introduced. These were antigens that, contradicting her mothers assertion, Jane had previously encountered and for which she had developed a secondary immune response. Reintroduction of the insect proteins caused an immediate inflammatory reaction that brought all the elements of the immune system to the site of the injury in order to remove the antigen.

The IgE-induced inflammation is an activity much like the inflammatory functions of complement. Many of the same elements of the inflammatory response are brought into action by both of these warning systems. The mechanism initiating the inflammation is different in each system; however, both result in the degranulation of mast cells. In the IgE system, antigen cross-links IgE antibody on the mast cell surface to degranulate the mast cell. In the complement system, antigen activates the system to produce the anaphylatoxin C3a, which degranulates mast cells.

A second function that has been identified for IgE reactions is the ability to provide immunologic protection against helminths and other parasites. The eosinophils, which arrive at the inflammatory site late in the response, contain a toxic major basic protein in their cytoplasmic granules that effectively kills these parasites.

New Vocabulary

A new vocabulary is associated with reactions of the IgE system. This vocabulary originated with studies of allergic responses that paralleled the investigation of other immune reactions. Because allergies and other IgE reactions are common occurrences, it is necessary to be familiar with both sets of nomenclature. Table 11-2 should help to familiarize the terms used to describe allergic reactions.

◀ **TABLE 11-2**
Vocabulary Associated with IgE Response

Term	Definition
Atopy	An inherited predisposition to respond to antigens with IgE antibodies
Atopic	An individual who responds to antigens with IgE antibodies
Anaphylaxis	Initially implies a hyperresponse to a toxin challenge, usually IgE mediated (i.e., the opposite of protection); unlike atopy, it does not imply an inherited predisposition
Allergen	Antigen that induces an IgE response
Sensitization	Immunization with or exposure to antigen that results in an IgE response
Reagin	IgE (reaginic antibody)

TWO PHASES OF THE IgE RESPONSE

Jane's response to the insect bite clearly indicated two phases that were separated by time. The first phase is the immediate response, followed by the second phase or slow reactions of anaphylaxis. Both phases result from IgE reacting with antigen and are secondary immune responses to the antigen.

Immediate Anaphylactic Response

The immediate anaphylactic response can be mimicked by the inflammatory mediator, *histamine*. For the immediate response to occur, antigen must stimulate mast cells to release the contents of their cytoplasmic granules. Major components of the granule contents are the vasoactive amines, which include histamine.

The IgE antibody is often referred to as a *cytophilic* (cell loving) antibody. Newly synthesized IgE antibody is rapidly bound to mast cells or circulating basophils via a high-affinity Fc_ε receptor on the mast cell or basophil surface. The affinity of this interaction is extremely high, and essentially all of the IgE is cell bound. Only a very small fraction of the total IgE antibody is detectable in the serum pool. Most of the IgE is present on the surfaces of circulating basophils and tissue-fixed mast cells (Fig. 11-2).

In Jane's response, because of previous antigen exposure, a relatively high proportion of the IgE antibodies that were bound to the mast-cell surface were specific for the insect antigen. Administration of antigen cross-links the membrane-bound IgE molecules. Cross-linking IgE molecules by antigen or by other methods that cross-link the Fc_ε receptors results in the rapid loss of the mast cell's prominent granules (Fig. 11-3). In this degranulation process the contents of the granules are expelled from the mast cell or basophil. The granule contents contain preformed mediators of anaphylaxis (Table 11-3). The most prominent preformed mediator is histamine.

Histamine Actions. Histamine and the other preformed mediators have dramatic activities that affect capillary permeability. The capillaries constrict, blood pressure increases, and vascular permeability increases, resulting in the net flow of fluid from the circulation into the interstitial spaces. As a result of this initial rapid response, the affected tissue is supplied with serum proteins, including antibody, complement, and clotting factors (see Fig. 11-3). Components of the immune system are available to respond rapidly to the antigen insult.

Other primary mediators are two important chemotactic factors: (1) the neutrophil

FIGURE 11-2

Function of IgE Antibody. *IgE antibodies are cytophilic. They bind to high-affinity Fc receptors on the surface of mast cells and circulating basophils. The antibodies function as a method to sensitize these cell types to antigen. The presence of antigen allows the cell-bound antibodies to be cross-linked, and the cell then releases its granule contents and begins synthesizing a series of secondary mediators. Any manipulations that can cross-link the Fc_ε receptor trigger the same response.*

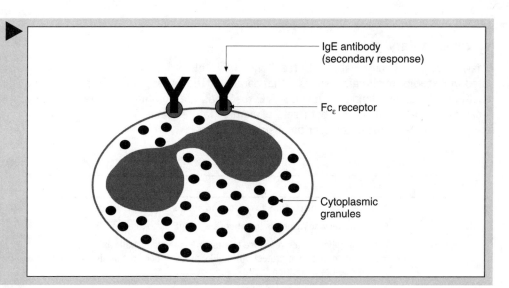

FIGURE 11-3

Immediate Anaphylactic Reaction. *The contents of the mast cell or basophil granules are responsible for the immediate anaphylactic reaction. They contain several important immediate mediators that play key roles in the rapid reaction. The granule contents include histamine and other vasoactive amines that increase capillary permeability and smooth muscle contraction. The chemotactic factors initially promote the accumulation of neutrophils and eventually promote the accumulation of eosinophils. The proteases and other hydrolases damage cellular structures, but they also help activate the complement and clotting systems.*

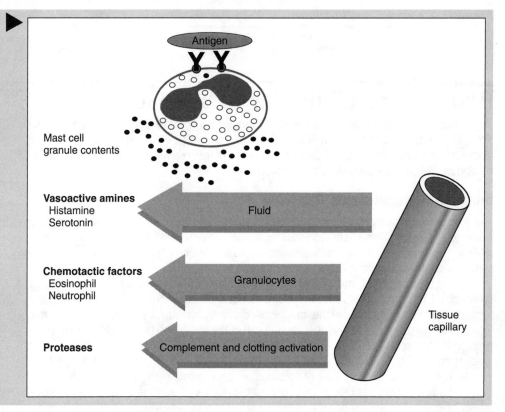

chemotactic factor of anaphylaxis (NCF-A) promotes an initial rapid infiltration of neutrophils, and (2) the eosinophil chemotactic factor of anaphylaxis (ECF-A) results in the eosinophil infiltration of the inflammatory site that occurs later in the response.

Secondary Anaphylactic Response

Following the kinetics of the response to the insect bite, it is clear that, in addition to the rapid reactions, there were equally important and dramatic slower responses. The slow reactions of anaphylaxis are under the control of a set of cell products produced by the stimulated (degranulated) mast cell. These cell products include both cytokines and lipid mediators of inflammation. A list of the major mast cell–synthesized and basophil-synthesized secondary inflammatory mediators is provided in Table 11-4.

◀ **TABLE 11-3**
Primary Mediators of Anaphylaxis

Class	Mediator	Activity
Vasoactive amine	Histamine	Smooth muscle contraction and increased vascular permeability
	Serotonin	Smooth muscle contraction and increased vascular permeability
Chemotactic factors	NCF-A	Neutrophil chemotaxis
	ECF-A	Eosinophil chemotaxis
Granule enzymes	Protease	Degradation of cellular components and activation of complement

Note. NCF-A = neutrophil chemotactic factor of anaphylaxis; ECF-A = eosinophil chemotactic factor of anaphylaxis.

◀ **TABLE 11-4**
Secondary Mediators of Anaphylaxis

Class	Mediator	Activity
Lipid mediators	Platelet-activating factor	Platelet aggregation, pulmonary smooth muscle contraction, and leukocyte activation
	Leukotrienes (SRS-A)	Pulmonary smooth muscle contraction and increased vascular permeability
	Prostaglandins	Pulmonary smooth muscle contraction and vasodilation
Peptides	Bradykinin	Smooth muscle contraction and increased vascular permeability
Cytokines	IL-1 and TNF	Inflammatory response
	IL-4	Promotes IgE isotype switch
	IL-5	Activates eosinophils
	Various other cytokines	

Note. SRS-A = slow-reacting substances of anaphylaxis; IL = interleukin; TNF = tumor necrosis factor.

The secondary mediators include cytokines such as interleukin-1 (IL-1), IL-4, and IL-5. These inflammatory cytokines, usually considered when discussing antigen presentation to CD4 helper T lymphocytes, are also produced by activated mast cells. A function of IL-5 not previously discussed but relevant to anaphylactic reactions is its ability to activate the eosinophil.

In addition to the synthesis and release of the cytokines, degranulation of mast cells also activates the enzyme phospholipase A_2 and initiates the synthesis of a series of lipid mediators of inflammation (Fig. 11-4). Many of these lipid mediators, such as prostaglandin D_2/(PGD_2), leukotriene C_4/(LTC_4), and platelet-activating factor (PAF), possess extremely potent activities that are similar to the activities described for histamine and prolong the histamine-like responses. Other prostaglandins express potent chemotactic activities for inflammatory cells. The student should be cautioned that not all mast cells are identical. Mast cells found in different tissues each produce their own unique set of lipid mediators. Consequently, the character of the slow reaction in different tissues can be slightly different.

The secondary anaphylactic mediators promote a cellular infiltration to the site of the response (Fig. 11-5). The cells entering the tissues initially include polymorphonuclear phagocytes in response to NCF-A. This is rapidly followed by a lymphocyte and monocyte accumulation, and as a result of ECF-A, there is an abundance of eosinophils in tissues, following mast cell degranulation.

*Prior to the chemical elucidation of their structure, the lipid mediators of anaphylaxis were called the **slow-reacting substances of anaphylaxis (SRS-A)**. This term is still commonly used.*

FIGURE 11-4 ▶

Synthesis of Lipid Mediators of Inflammation. *Degranulation of the mast cell or basophil also alters cellular metabolism and begins the synthesis of a series of secondary mediators. One class of secondary mediators is the arachidonic acid metabolites. Mast cell degranulation activates the enzyme phospholipase A$_2$, which acts on the cell membrane to hydrolyze arachidonic acid, from the phospholipid structure. In addition, cyclooxygenase and lipoxygenases are activated, which begins the synthesis of the prostaglandins and leukotrienes. These compounds are extremely potent vasodilators and promote the contraction of pulmonary smooth muscle.*

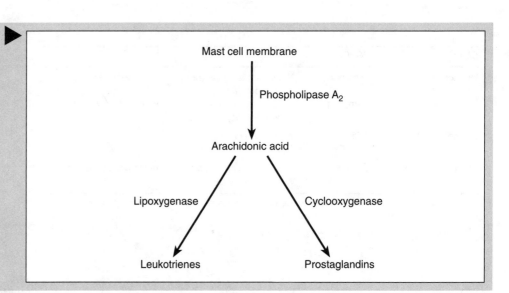

FIGURE 11-5 ▶

Secondary Anaphylactic Reactions. *The secondary or synthesized mediators of anaphylaxis continue the inflammatory response that was initiated by the immediate reaction. The lipid mediators prolong the histamine-like reactions of smooth muscle–contraction vasodilation. Numerous cytokines are also synthesized and released during the second phase of the reaction. Cytokines like interleukin-1 (IL-1) and tumor necrosis factor possess the activities that promote cell-mediated inflammation with the infiltration of lymphocytes and monocytes into the site. IL-4 helps direct isotype switching to the IgE isotype, and IL-5, having multiple stimulatory activities, also activates the eosinophils that are brought to the inflammatory site by the eosinophil chemotactic factor.*

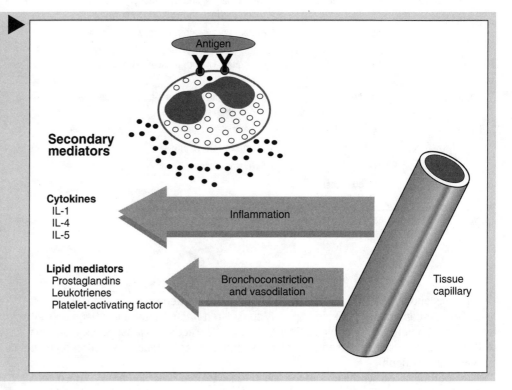

Eosinophil Functions. The eosinophil, a later arrival at the anaphylactic site, has critical functions that have not, as yet, been discussed in depth. Two distinct characteristics of eosinophils give clues to their functional role in the anaphylactic response, and these functions are based on their granule contents.

Eosinophil granules have a potent histaminase, an enzyme that converts histamine to inactive products. This enzyme plays a functional role in the detoxification of the histamine released by the immediate reaction of anaphylaxis and helps to regulate, thereby lessening, anaphylactic responses. A second critical function of the eosinophil resides in the major basic protein that is found in the cytoplasmic granules. The major basic protein of the eosinophil granule is toxic to both foreign and autologous cells. When directed to a foreign cell or organism (e.g., helminth) by antibody targeting, the major basic protein has the potential to kill the target organism. However, when continually released as the result of chronic anaphylactic reactions (e.g., asthma), the major basic protein can be responsible for a considerable amount of the tissue damage to normal tissues that is associated with chronic IgE stimulation.

REGULATION OF IgE SYNTHESIS

What controls the extent of IgE production, and why do we not react to antigen using other immunologic methods (e.g., IgG, IgA, delayed-type hypersensitivity [DTH] reactions)? To understand the relationship between different types of inflammatory responses, it is necessary to understand the mutual regulation of the helper T cells, Th1 and Th2. The cytokine interferon-γ, synthesized by the Th1 cells, has a potent suppressive activity on Th2 cell function in addition to mediating DTH reactions. Conversely, the cytokines IL-4 and IL-10 from activated Th2 cells enhance IgE isotype switching and suppress Th1 cell functions, respectively. The type of immune response observed is a direct result of this balance between the factors activating Th1 and Th2 cell types. At present, it is difficult to understand fully all of the factors that determine whether someone will have an allergic response to antigen or respond to the same antigen with either an IgG, IgA, or DTH response. There are, however, certain criteria that tend to promote IgE reactions. In addition to the unknown environmental factors that can alter the activity balance of Th1 and Th2, host genetics play a major role in allowing IgE responses. Also, certain types of antigens and routes of antigen exposure promote IgE reactions. Moreover, selective deficiency of the IgA immune response puts an individual at significantly increased risk for IgE-mediated reactions.

> **Known Factors That Promote IgE Response**
> - *Host genetics*
> - *Antigen characteristics*
> - *Route and history of antigen exposure*
> - *Unknown environmental factors that increase amounts or activity of Th2 cytokines relative to Th1 cytokines*

RESOLUTION OF CLINICAL CASE

When the insect bit Jane, it left some of its protein in the wound. This was not the first time that Jane had been exposed to the antigen. On first exposure, Jane developed an IgE immune response to the insect protein. Because of genetics, the route of the antigen administration, and other unknown environmental factors, the B lymphocytes responding to the insect antigen were given the information necessary to induce a switch to the IgE isotype. On second exposure to the antigen, the IgE product of the primary response was on the surface of the tissue mast cells. Reintroduction of the antigen cross-linked the mast cell–bound IgE antibody, stimulating mast cell degranulation. The histamine, along with other preformed mediators, increased vascular permeability and smooth muscle contraction, eventually leading to the initial edematous wheal and flair. Degranulation was also accompanied by the synthesis of several secondary factors, including cytokines and lipid mediators. The lipid mediators continued the histamine-like responses, and the cytokines promoted lymphocyte- and monocyte-mediated inflammatory responses. The result of these slower reactions was an indurated swelling characterized by monocytes, lymphocytes, and eosinophils. During this response, there was a significant amount of damage to healthy tissue. The damage was due not only to the tissue destruction associated with the cells and factors discussed above but also to the basic protein associated with the granule contents of the eosinophil, which collected at the inflammatory site. With the elimination of insect antigen, Jane's anaphylactic response eventually resolved, and the repair factors released from the monocytes eventually promoted increased fibroblast proliferation. However, in conditions where there is chronic activation of the IgE system, such as in chronic asthma, the damage to tissue is not easily controlled by antigen concentration, and there is continued inflammatory response, continued tissue damage, and continued fibrosis. Currently, there are multiple approaches to therapeutic intervention in this type of response. Some of these approaches, as well as methods still under investigation, are outlined in Fig. 11-6.

FIGURE 11-6 ▶

Summary of the IgE Response. *This figure outlines a summary of the cellular events that took place in Jane prior to or during her response to the insect antigen. There are multiple approaches for the eventual therapeutic intervention in this cascade of events. Some of these approaches are in current use, such as blocking the actions of the primary and secondary mediators, avoiding the allergen, and inhibiting the binding of IgE to mast cells or preventing the mast cell stimulation. Other approaches are being actively investigated. Many of these include looking for ways to alter how the B cell receives signals from the helper T cell so that the effects of interleukin-4 are diminished and the selected B lymphocyte can respond with a different antibody isotype.*

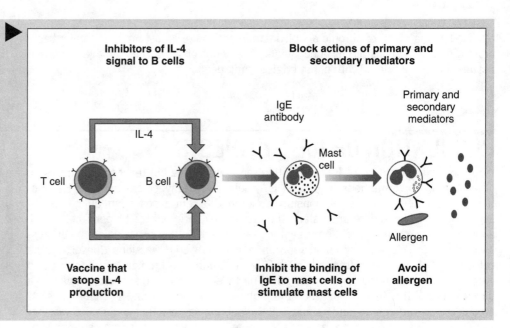

REVIEW QUESTIONS

Directions: For each of the following questions, choose the **one best** answer.

1. Which of the following explanations correctly characterizes the swelling associated with the immediate reaction of anaphylaxis?

    (A) There is lymphocyte accumulation in the tissue.

    (B) There is neutrophil accumulation in the tissue.

    (C) There is eosinophil accumulation in the tissue.

    (D) There is an initial neutrophil accumulation, followed by lymphocytes, monocytes, and eosinophils in the tissue.

    (E) The initial swelling is unrelated to an accumulation of inflammatory cells.

2. Which of the following mediators is primarily responsible for the initial rapid reaction of anaphylaxis?

    (A) Histamine

    (B) ECF-A

    (C) Prostaglandin

    (D) Leukotriene

    (E) IL-1

3. Exceedingly low serum concentrations of IgE reflect which of the following conditions?

    (A) The minor role played by IgE-mediated reactions

    (B) The low IgE synthetic rate

    (C) The high rate of turnover (synthesis and loss) of the IgE antibody

    (D) The infrequent nature of IgE reactions

    (E) The high-affinity binding to mast cells and basophils

4. A patient suffered a severe anaphylactic response to a therapeutic dose of penicillin. Which of the following is the correct interpretation of this response?

    (A) The patient had been exposed previously to penicillin.

    (B) This was the patient's first exposure to penicillin.

    (C) The patient will also exhibit allergies and other IgE reactions.

    (D) The patient has a defect in the IgG system, which allowed the IgE response.

    (E) An allergic reaction to penicillin is not immunologically mediated.

5. Which of the following mast cell factors is a secondary or delayed mediator of anaphylaxis?

    (A) Histamine

    (B) Serotonin

    (C) ECF-A

    (D) NCF-A

    (E) IL-5

Note. Abbreviations used in the questions: ECF-A = eosinophil chemotactic factor of anaphylaxis; IL-1 = interleukin-1; IgE = immunoglobulin E; IgG = immunoglobulin G; NCF-A = neutrophil chemotactic factor of anaphylaxis; IL-5 = interleukin-5; DTH = delayed-type hypersensitivity.

6. Which of the following events directly causes the degranulation of mast cells?

   (A) Activation of complement via the alternate pathway

   (B) DTH reactions

   (C) CD8 reactions

   (D) Macrophage activation by IL-1

   (E) IgE binding to the mast cell surface

7. Which of the following best describes the role of eosinophils in anaphylactic responses?

   (A) Since the eosinophil arrives late in the anaphylactic reaction, it has no role in the response.

   (B) Eosinophils are the cellular source of histamine, which causes the immediate reaction.

   (C) The eosinophil is the cellular source of the lipid mediators of anaphylaxis.

   (D) The major basic protein contained in eosinophil granules causes some of the tissue damage associated with atopic reactions.

   (E) Eosinophils are circulating cells and are not found in the tissues.

8. Immediately upon receiving a blood transfusion, a patient began experiencing allergic reactions to penicillin. This new reaction is best explained by which of the following?

   (A) The blood used for the transfusion was contaminated with penicillin.

   (B) The reaction is most probably not immunologic in nature.

   (C) This is an example of passive immunization.

   (D) Because of the low concentration of IgE in serum, this reaction can only be due to an IgG response.

9. Which of the following would be the best reagent to inhibit selectively IgE-mediated reactions?

   (A) An agent that prevents IgE from binding to mast cells

   (B) An agent that inhibits CD4-cell function

   (C) An agent that inhibits B-cell differentiation

   (D) An agent that inhibits all histamine functions

10. An inhibitor of cyclooxygenase would be expected to have which of the following effects on an anaphylactic response?

    (A) Prevent mast cell degranulation

    (B) Alter the IgE synthetic rate

    (C) Interfere with the biologic functions of histamine

    (D) Prevent eosinophil chemotaxis

    (E) Decrease effects of the secondary lipid mediators of anaphylaxis

ANSWERS AND EXPLANATIONS

1. **The answer is E.** The immediate reaction of anaphylaxis is due primarily to the actions of histamine, which causes vasodilation and vascular constriction. The result is fluid build-up in the area of the antigen that is essentially cell free. Following this initial reaction, a cellular infiltration of the site is observed. There is a transient increase in neutrophils, which are rapidly replaced by lymphocytes, monocytes, and eosinophils.

2. **The answer is A.** Almost all of the events of the immediate reaction can be mimicked by histamine. Chemotactic factors are also included in some of the preformed mediators of anaphylaxis contained in the granules. However, their effect is only observed after cells have had time to migrate to the inflammatory site. The other compounds listed are mediators of the slow reactions.

3. **The answer is E.** IgE is a cytophilic antibody, which means that it is rapidly bound to mast cells and basophils. Estimates of the IgE synthetic rate are much higher than can be accounted for by the low serum concentration. Moreover, although the serum half-life of IgE is relatively rapid, the half-life of an IgE molecule bound to the mast cell surface is significantly longer.

4. **The answer is A.** IgE reactions are secondary immune responses and require an initial exposure to the antigen before the anaphylactic response is observed. Anaphylactic reactions are, like other immune reactions, antigen specific, and an allergic response to one antigen does not necessarily mean that the individual will exhibit IgE responses to all antigens. Atopic individuals, however, have a propensity to respond with the IgE system.

5. **The answer is E.** IL-5, which is normally considered a lymphokine associated with CD4 lymphocytes, is also synthesized by degranulated mast cells and basophils. The activated mast cell synthesizes a variety of cytokines that potentially can alter future immune responses to promote an IgE isotype switch. All remaining choices are preformed mediators of anaphylaxis.

6. **The answer is A.** Activation of complement by either the alternate or classic pathway results in the generation of C3 convertase, which catalyzes the cleavage of C3 into C3a and C3b. C3a, in addition to some of the other small peptide fragments from complement activation, is a potent anaphylatoxin. Anaphylatoxins degranulate mast cells and basophils as does the cross-linking of mast cell–bound IgE. IgE is normally bound to the surface of mast cells and basophils. Simply binding IgE to the surface of the mast cell will not degranulate the cell. Degranulation requires cross-linking the Fc_ε receptors.

7. **The answer is D.** Although the eosinophil arrives late in the response, it plays major roles in both the protection against antigen and the associated tissue damage of the response. The eosinophil granules contain histaminase, which can potentially down-regulate histamine responses. Moreover, the granules contain a major basic protein that is cytotoxic both to viable antigens and normal tissues.

8. **The answer is C.** Anaphylactic reactions are IgE mediated. In the scenario presented in this question, the IgE antibody (transfusion) that was administered can be rapidly bound to the mast cell or basophil surface. If the administered IgE is rich in antibody to a specific antigen, the antibody can sensitize mast cells to react to the antigen. This type of passive immunity has been reported to last in excess of 3 months.

9. **The answer is A.** If IgE cannot bind to mast cells, both the immediate and delayed reactions of anaphylaxis cannot be initiated by the antibody response. Complement component C3a will still be able to effect mast cell degranulation. The other options result in a wide-ranging inhibition of inflammatory responses.

10. **The answer is E.** Cyclooxygenase is involved in the first step in the synthetic pathway leading to prostaglandins. Inhibition of this enzyme decreases the amount of prostaglandin synthesized following a challenge with an allergen. Inhibition of cyclooxygenase will not inhibit immediate reactions or the synthesis of other mediators of the delayed anaphylactic reaction.

12

MUCOSAL IMMUNITY

CHAPTER OUTLINE

INTRODUCTION OF CLINICAL CASE

Johnny Larson, a 4-year-old, was brought to his family practice physician by his parents because they were concerned about his slow growth. The main complaint, however, was the relatively high frequency of loose stools. Upon examination, it became apparent that Johnny was not growing at the expected rate and exhibited symptoms that suggested malabsorption problems. Laboratory analysis showed anemia, confirmed vitamin deficiencies, and revealed a marked elevation in the serum level of immunoglobulin A (IgA).

ROLE AND MAGNITUDE OF THE IgA RESPONSE

Although the laboratory analysis showed that Johnny was suffering from several nutritional deficiencies, the elevated level of IgA was an unexpected finding. IgA is the antibody isotype normally found in the secretory sites. When considering daily synthetic rate, IgA, of all antibody isotypes, is the major immunoglobulin. It has been estimated that almost 70% of the immunoglobulin synthesized per day is the IgA isotype.

IgA protects mucosal sites using mechanisms that are different from those described for the other antibody isotypes. The antibody has not been convincingly demonstrated to activate the complement system or to bind Fc-receptor-bearing cytotoxic cells. IgA protects mucosal sites by

> **IgA Protective Mechanisms**
> • *Prevent bacterial colonization*
> • *Inhibit viral adherence*
> • *Block the activity of biologic toxins*
> • *Limit the absorption of macromolecular antigens*

binding to bacterial and viral pathogens and preventing their colonization and adherence. IgA antibodies can also bind active sites of some toxic proteins and inactivate or block their toxic activity. Probably one of the most significant functions of the IgA system is the role that it plays in the gut, where it binds macromolecular antigens and prevents their absorption. This activity limits subsequent immunoglobulin G (IgG), immunoglobulin E (IgE), and delayed-type hypersensitivity (DTH) immune responses that would result from the exposure.

Clearly, one of the critical properties the IgA molecule has is sufficient physical and chemical stability to survive the conditions found in the mucosal sites. An even more stringent limitation is that the IgA response must be initiated and controlled independently from other immune responses. Successful protection of mucosal sites requires the gut immune system to activate the IgA response selectively and simultaneously suppress DTH and antibody responses of the IgG and IgE isotypes. In this context, it is as if the IgA system is a totally separate immune system. Early observations about mucosal immunity demonstrated a reciprocal relationship between serum antibody and mucosal antibody: when there was an elevated serum antibody response, the mucosal response was diminished, and when there was an elevated mucosal response, the serum response was diminished. Johnny's problem does not stem from an immunodeficiency or lack of an immune response. Johnny's problem is that, instead of making an IgA response, he is mounting an inappropriate type of immune response to gluten (gliadin), a protein found in wheat, oats, and barley.

*The active secretory IgA immune response associated with diminished IgG, IgE, and DTH reactions has given rise to the term **oral tolerance**, which implies that, by immunizing the secretory immune system, it is possible to prevent or tolerate other systemic immune responses to the same antigen. Oral tolerance is being investigated as one method to regulate immune responses in an antigen-specific manner.*

IgA MOLECULE: RELATIONSHIP OF STRUCTURE TO FUNCTION

The IgA molecule comes in three distinctly different configurations. Two structures of the IgA molecules are found in serum, and the third structure is limited to the mucosal secretions. The three different types of IgA include the monomer, the dimer, and a secretory form of the dimer.

The monomeric form of the IgA molecule has a structure that is essentially identical to the generic immunoglobulin. The α heavy chain is slightly larger, with a higher carbohydrate content. The molecule, however, still follows the generic pattern of two α heavy chains and two light chains (either κ or λ).

In addition to the monomeric IgA molecule, there is a dimeric version. In the dimer, the Fc portions of two monomeric IgA molecules are held together by a joining (J) chain. This is the same J chain that is found in the other polymeric immunoglobulin, IgM. The monomeric and dimeric molecules found in serum are not present in secretions.

The third form of the IgA molecule is associated with an additional polypeptide chain called *secretory component*. Secretory component is a 70,000-dalton, highly glycosylated protein that provides the IgA molecule with the protease resistance it requires to function in the harsh environment of the mucosal sites. Table 12-1 compares the physical and chemical properties of the three IgA molecules.

TABLE 12-1
Physical and Chemical Properties of IgA

	Monomeric IgA	Dimeric IgA	Secretory IgA
Sedimentation coefficient	8s	10s	11s
Location	Serum	Serum	Mucosal sites
Antibody composition			
α chains	2	4	4
Light chains	2	4	4
Joining chain	—	1	1
Secretory component	—	—	1

Note. s = sedimentation constant expressed in Svedberg units.

ANATOMY OF THE IgA SYSTEM

The secretory immune system can be viewed as composed of two different types of tissues that are separate from the spleen, lymph nodes, and other lymphatic tissues necessary for IgG, IgE, and DTH responses. These tissues are the organized and the diffuse mucosal lymphoid tissues.

Organized Lymphoid Tissues

Throughout mucosal sites, there are aggregates of lymphoid tissue. The Peyer's patches found in the intestine are an example of this organized structure. Other examples include the tonsils and appendix, as well as multiple other lymphoid aggregates. All mucosal sites contain this organized lymphoid tissue. However, the best studied are the Peyer's patches of the gut. Fig. 12-1 schematically illustrates the cellular organization of the tissue. At the interface between the gut lumen and the organized lymphoid tissue, there is an area that protrudes into the lumen and lacks the villous structure of the intestinal border. This structure is often referred to as the dome of a Peyer's patch. One type of cell, the M cell, is prominent in the dome area and on the epithelial surface. The M cell is phagocytic, but it lacks the granular structures of most antigen-presenting cells (APCs) and is deficient in lysosomal enzymes. Therefore, the M cell cannot effectively process or present the phagocytized antigen in the context of the class II major histocompatibility complex (MHC) molecule. The M cell's role is that of an antigen-pumping cell. It primarily transfers particulate antigen from the lumen of the secretory site into the dome area of the organized lymphoid tissue. Underneath the M-cell layer is an aggregation of B cells, T cells, and APCs. When the antigen is introduced into this area, lymphocytes can be clonally selected. Antigen samples will be phagocytized by the resident monocytes and presented to CD4 T cells. All of the events that take place in either the lymph node or spleen happen locally in the dome area of the organized mucosal lymphoid tissues. The antigen-selected cells receive help and begin proliferating, and they eventually develop into a primary lymphoid follicle in the same manner that antigen selection happens in the lymph node or the spleen.

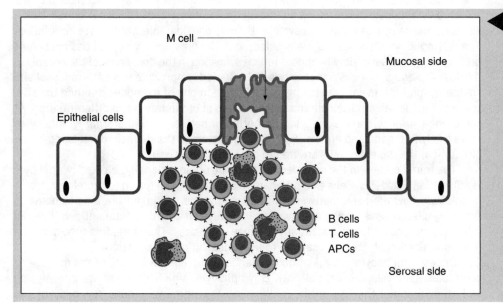

FIGURE 12-1

Organized Lymphoid Tissue. *Throughout the mucosal sites, there are aggregations of lymphoid tissue, in which there are the organized lymphoid tissues represented by the Peyer's patches of the intestine. The organized tissue consists of a dome of cells that protrudes into the intestinal lumen. A prominent cell in this dome is an M cell. Although it has a low granule content, the M cell is phagocytic and transports antigen across the epithelial layer of cells. In the dome area, the antigen encounters B lymphocytes, T lymphocytes, and antigen-presenting cells (APCs). All of the cellular components necessary to begin an immune response are present in the area of the mucosal lymphoid aggregates.*

Diffuse Lymphoid Tissues

The *mucosal-associated lymphoid tissue (MALT)* not only refers to the *gut-associated lymphoid tissues (GALT)* but includes the *bronchial-associated lymphoid tissues (BALT)* and the lymphoid tissues found at all secretory sites.

The second type of mucosal lymphoid tissue is the diffuse mucosal lymphoid tissue (Fig. 12-2). At each of the secretory sites, lymphocytes (B cells, T cells), monocytes, and IgA-producing plasma cells can be identified in the lamina propria layer. In addition, lymphocytes can be seen in the epithelial tissues and the submucosal layers. The entire mucosal site, then, can be considered the diffuse mucosal lymphoid tissue, and it supports antibody production. Taken together, the organized and diffuse mucosal lymphoid tissues comprise a significant portion of the entire immune system.

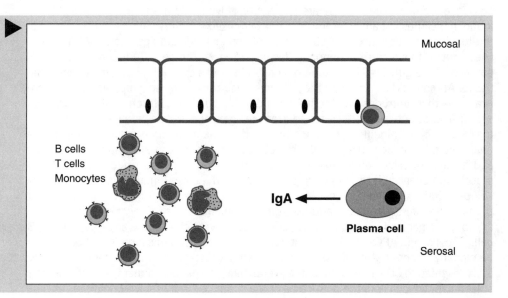

FIGURE 12-2

Diffuse Lymphoid Tissue. *Lymphoid cells are found scattered throughout the lamina propria of the mucosal sites. Lymphocytes can also be found in the submucosal layers and even between epithelial cells. B cells, T cells, macrophages, and importantly, plasma cells are all found in this area. The primary antibody isotype secreted by the plasma cells is IgA. Because of the number of lymphocytes found there, all secretory sites should be considered major lymphoid organs.*

LYMPHOCYTE CIRCULATION

For the generation of an IgG antibody response, the proliferation and maturation of the selected lymphocyte takes place in the germinal centers of the local lymph node. However, in the mucosal immune system, there is considerable lymphocyte circulation. The B lymphocyte that was originally selected in the organized lymphoid tissues begins proliferating, and secondary lymphoid follicles develop in the dome area of the organized tissues. The daughter cells from the original selected lymphocyte leave the mucosal site via the lymphatics, eventually taking up residence in one of the nodes draining the site. In the node, the selected cell continues its process of proliferation and differentiation. At some point prior to completing its differentiation pathway, the maturing lymphocytes leave the lymph node and enter the circulatory system at the thoracic duct. Once in the circulation, the daughter cells are free to circulate to all tissues.

The traffic pattern of the cells derived from the original clonally selected lymphocyte is outlined in Fig. 12-3. Cells that originate in a secretory site return to secretory sites. It is unknown how the cells that were initially stimulated in the gut are able to home to secretory sites. This is clearly an advantage because an environmental antigen that can infect one mucosal site can potentially colonize other sites. Therefore, this system allows the immunization of one mucosal site to immunize all mucosal sites.

Once a lymphocyte has taken up residence in the lamina propria of the mucosa, it completes its developmental pathway. B lymphocytes finally differentiate into plasma cells that produce the IgA antibody. Whereas the primary immune response of the mucosa (outlined above) includes a significant amount of lymphocyte traffic, the secondary response to a mucosal antigen is rapid and can remain local. In this case, the memory B lymphocytes that are stimulated with antigen immediately begin producing and secreting IgA antibody.

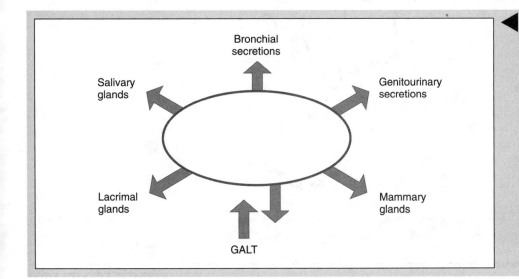

◀ FIGURE 12-3
Lymphocyte Circulation. *When a lymphocyte has been selected in the organized lymphoid tissues, it begins proliferating, initially in the organized lymphoid tissue itself and then in the local lymph node. Eventually, the daughter cells leave the node and enter the circulation via the thoracic duct. Once in the circulation, the daughter cells can home to all of the secretory sites and colonize those sites. This system allows an antigen to immunize via one specific mucosal site, and the resulting immune response protects all mucosal sites. GALT = gut-associated lymphoid tissue.*

TRANSPORT OF IgA INTO THE MUCOSAL FLUIDS

The IgA-producing plasma cells in the mucosa make both the monomeric (8*s*) and dimeric (10*s*) forms of the molecule. There are two potential fates for this IgA. Both the 8*s* and 10*s* IgA molecules can diffuse through the interstitial space and eventually enter the circulation. In Johnny, serum levels of IgA were significantly elevated. The serum IgA had its origin in mucosal sites, and the elevated level indicates there is an active immune response happening in the mucosal site. In addition to the mucosal contribution to the serum IgA pool, IgA is synthesized in the bone marrow. The origin of this bone marrow pool is not clear. The biologic role of the serum IgA also is not clear. The serum molecule has a potential regulatory function in limiting antigen that is available to induce other immune responses, and in some species, the 10*s* form of the serum IgA molecule can be used by the liver for the removal of circulating antigen.

The major fate of the 10*s* IgA molecule, however, is its secretion into the lumen of the mucosal site. IgA is transported into the lumen by an IgA-specific system that selectively binds the 10*s* IgA molecule and transports it across the epithelial cell (Fig. 12-4). On the serosal surface of the epithelial cell layer is a receptor specific for the Fc portion of the dimeric IgA molecule (Fc$_\alpha$ receptor). When the receptor binds the 10*s* IgA molecule, a covalent (disulfide) bond is formed between the receptor and the IgA molecule. This IgA receptor complex is then internalized by the epithelial cell and transported across the cell, where it is expressed on the mucosal surface. On the mucosal surface, both the IgA and the covalently attached receptor are removed from the cell by proteolysis. The secreted form of IgA contains the remnants of the Fc$_\alpha$ receptor and is now called secretory component. The secretory component–IgA complex (11*s* IgA or secretory IgA) provides the molecule with the increased chemical and proteolytic stability necessary to function in the mucosal environment. Once in the mucosal environment, the antibody can bind antigen and prevent colonization, inhibit adherence, and limit absorption of macromolecular antigens.

FIGURE 12-4 ▶

IgA Transport. *The plasma cells in the diffuse mucosal tissues produce both 8s and 10s IgA. These antibodies can diffuse into the circulation. The 10s IgA, however, is also bound to a specific Fcα receptor on the serosal face of the epithelial cell. The IgA-receptor complex is transported to the mucosal face of the cell and eventually expressed on the mucosal surface. The IgA-receptor complex is then released from the mucosal surface by proteolysis in such a way that the mucosal form of IgA is found with the receptor attached. The secreted form of IgA with the attached receptor is 11s in size, and the receptor is now called secretory component.*

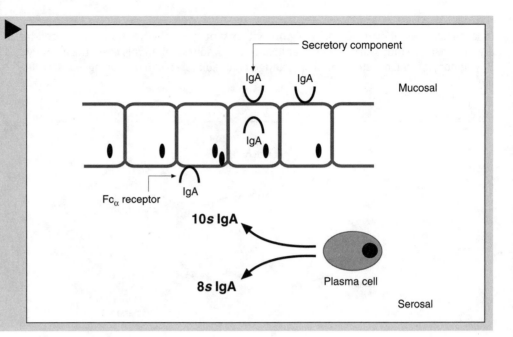

IgA DEFICIENCY

Most common of all immunodeficiency syndromes, selective deficiency in IgA production, affects approximately 1 in 700 individuals. The disorder appears to be the result of an inability to secrete the IgA molecule rather than an arrested development of the IgA system. There is considerable discussion about the impact of this deficiency on an individual's health. Some investigators consider IgA deficiency to be of minor significance because other immune mechanisms can compensate for the loss of IgA function; yet, other investigators associate IgA deficiencies with recurrent sinopulmonary infections, allergies, gastrointestinal tract disease, and autoimmune disease. In spite of the controversy, it is clear that IgA-deficient individuals are at increased risk for transfusion reaction brought about by the IgA content of normal serum. To prevent these reactions, stocks of IgA-deficient serum and blood are maintained specifically for IgA-deficient individuals.

There is a second form of IgA deficiency, however, that is even more common. This is a transient IgA deficiency, which takes place during development. Fig. 12-5 charts the development of the humoral immune system during the first year of an infant's life. From this figure, it is clear that different antibody isotypes develop at different rates. IgM and IgG responses develop early, during the first year of life, whereas the IgA system matures far more slowly. The role that this differential development plays in future health issues for the child is controversial and extremely difficult to evaluate accurately.

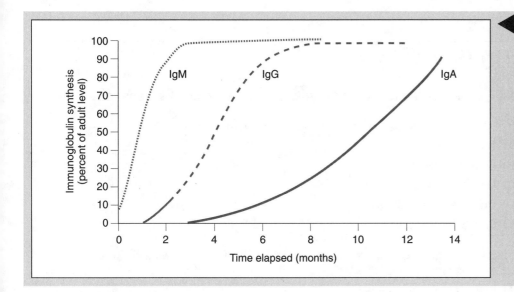

FIGURE 12-5
IgA Ontogeny. *Isotype responses of the humoral immune system develop at different rates. IgM is the earliest of the isotypes to develop. In cases where there has been an intrauterine infection, the IgM response at birth can be quite significant. The IgM response is followed, chronologically, by the IgG response. The last isotype to develop is IgA.*

RESOLUTION OF CLINICAL CASE

A biopsy of Johnny's intestinal mucosal surface showed a significant amount of damage. There was a loss of the villi, which accounted for the malabsorption. The intestinal crypts were measurably elongated, indicating a significant amount of cell proliferation in response to the injury, and in the tissue there was a massive lymphocyte infiltration. The results of the biopsy indicated that Johnny had an immune response to gluten. However, in Johnny's case, the response and tissue damage were not attributable to the IgA isotype but instead to other immune mechanisms. Upon each exposure to products containing gluten, the cell-mediated and humopral immune responses recruited and activated additional inflammatory cells and was responsible for the damage to the intestinal epthelium associated with removing the gluten antigens. Because of the damaged intestinal surface, the intestinal contents as well as macromolecules, bacteria, and virus can all infect the patient and initiate multiple inflammatory reactions, including new or enhanced IgA reactions. To avoid these problems in the future, Johnny needs to avoid the gluten antigens.

Johnny suffers from gluten enteropathy or celiac sprue. He primarily responds to the gluten antigens with IgG antibody. However, patients can present with a variety of signs and symptoms that reflect the activities of other immune responses.

REVIEW QUESTIONS

Directions: For each of the following questions, choose the **one best** answer.

1. Which of the following is the major site of immunoglobulin A (IgA) production?
    (A) Lymph node
    (B) Spleen
    (C) Liver
    (D) Organized mucosal tissue
    (E) Diffuse mucosal tissue

2. IgA effects protection against an antigen using which of the following biologic effector mechanisms of antibodies?
    (A) Binding to Fc killer cells
    (B) Opsonization
    (C) Fixation of complement
    (D) Limiting absorption and adsorption
    (E) Activating delayed-type hypersensitivity reactions

3. The polypeptide chains that comprise the final structure of secretory IgA (11s IgA) are derived from which type of cells?
    (A) Plasma cells
    (B) B cells
    (C) T cells
    (D) Epithelial cells
    (E) Plasma cells and epithelial cells

4. In the organized lymphoid tissue, which of the following best describes the M cell's function?
    (A) It is unrelated to the immune response.
    (B) It is that of an antigen-presenting cell (APC).
    (C) It provides the information that allows B lymphocytes to switch to IgA isotype.
    (D) It transports antigen across the epithelial layer.
    (E) It prevents antigen transport.

5. Which of the following statements correctly describes the fate of a B lymphocyte that has been selected in a mucosal site?
    (A) It immediately leaves the site and completes its developmental pathway in the lymph node.
    (B) After an initial proliferation in the organized mucosal tissue, the daughter cells leave the mucosal site and eventually enter the circulation. The daughter cells only home to the site of initial stimulation.
    (C) After an initial proliferation in the organized mucosal tissue, the daughter cells leave the mucosal site and eventually enter the circulation. The daughter cells can then populate any mucosal site.
    (D) Upon stimulation, the selected B lymphocyte remains at the mucosal site and develops into a plasma cell.

6. Which of the following is a correct description of the relative magnitude of the IgA response compared to other immune responses?

   (A) Serum antibody concentrations accurately reflect the immunoglobulin synthetic capacity for each of the isotypes.

   (B) The major antibody, in terms of daily synthetic rate, is IgA.

   (C) The major antibody, in terms of daily synthetic rate, is IgG.

   (D) The IgA daily synthetic rate is approximately equal to that of IgM.

7. Which of the following statements best describes the function of secretory component?

   (A) It stabilizes IgA against proteases.

   (B) It transports IgA across the epithelial cell layer.

   (C) It stabilizes IgA against proteases and transports it across the epithelial cell layer.

   (D) It neither stabilizes IgA against proteases nor transports it across the epithelial cell layer.

8. Which of the following correctly describes the diffuse mucosal lymphoid tissue?

   (A) It is a minor component of the immune system, best represented by the Peyer's patches found in the gut.

   (B) It refers only to the occasional B cell or plasma cell found in the lamina propria of the mucosal sites.

   (C) It comprises an extensive collection of B cells, T cells, macrophages, and plasma cells found at all mucosal sites.

   (D) It is an aggregation of lymphoid tissue found in the dome areas of Peyer's patches.

9. A selective IgA deficiency is best described by which of the following statements?

   (A) It is an extremely rare condition, which is manifested by continual mucosal infections.

   (B) It is an extremely rare condition, which is associated with increased mucosal infections, autoimmunity, allergic responses, and elevated responses to macromolecular antigens.

   (C) It is a relatively common condition, which is manifested by continual mucosal infections.

   (D) It is a relatively common condition, which may or may not be associated with overt symptoms of mucosal infections, autoimmunity, increased allergic responses, and elevated responses to macromolecular antigens.

10. Which of the following statements best describes the development of the IgA immune system?

   (A) IgA immune responses develop much later than immune responses for other isotypes.

   (B) IgA immune responses develop earlier than other immune responses.

   (C) The IgA system develops at about the same time as the IgG response.

   (D) The IgA antibody system does not develop until the first exposure to a mucosal antigen.

ANSWERS AND EXPLANATIONS

1. **The answer is E.** In the mucosal immune system, clonal selection takes place in the organized mucosal tissues, whereas antibody production is primarily found in the lamina propria of the secretory sites. Antibodies of other isotypes are also synthesized in the diffuse mucosal tissues, although at a significantly lower concentration.

2. **The answer is D.** The 11s IgA antibody prevents antigen access across mucosal sites. It does not appear to function with any other accessory cells or molecules. The functions of the 8s and 10s IgA molecules are not as clear.

3. **The answer is E.** IgA is an example of a single protein that is synthesized by two different cell types. The light, heavy, and joining chain portions of IgA are synthesized by the lamina propria plasma cell, whereas the secretory component is a part of the epithelial IgA transport mechanism and is synthesized by the epithelial cell.

4. **The answer is D.** The M cell is a phagocytic cell that is deficient in cytoplasmic granules. It appears to be related to other APCs, but it cannot process antigen. It transports antigen into the organized lymphoid structures.

5. **The answer is C.** The secretory immune system has the capacity to allow immunization of one mucosal site to provide immune protection at all secretory sites. After initial proliferation at the local site, daughter cells from the originally stimulated cell enter the circulation and seed the other sites.

6. **The answer is B.** Approximately 70% of the antibody made daily is the IgA isotype.

7. **The answer is C.** Secretory component is a multifunctional protein. Not only does it function as an epithelial-cell receptor for IgA, promoting the transport of IgA across the epithelial cell, but it also protects IgA against the harsh environmental conditions of the gut.

8. **The answer is C.** The mucosal tissues are rich in cells of the lymphatic system. The gut and other mucosal sites can be considered as major lymphoid organs.

9. **The answer is D.** Selective IgA deficiency is found in approximately 1 in 700 individuals. Although loss of IgA function would be expected to put an individual at risk for multiple infections and continual macromolecular antigen stimulation of the mucosal sites, other elements of both acquired immunity and natural immunity are still able to function. Consequently, IgA-deficient individuals may exhibit a variety of symptoms or have no detectable symptoms.

10. **The answer is A.** IgA is the last of the isotype responses to mature. This observation has led to several controversial theories. One suggests that early exposures to common antigens can induce responses that, later in life, lead to autoimmunity or other unexpected immune responses. Although interesting, this is a hypothesis that is extremely difficult to assess.

13 CELL-MEDIATED IMMUNITY

INTRODUCTION OF CLINICAL CASE

Michael, a 24-year-old applying for a position as a teacher at a local high school, was sent to see his physician because of a positive purified protein derivative (PPD) test that was part of his pre-employment physical. Michael admitted being abnormally tired recently. He had also experienced periods of being short of breath with some minor chest pains, and because of that, had curtailed his normal exercise routine. Michael remembered having had a cold several months ago, which seemed to hang on longer than usual and which was associated with a productive cough. He also said that he had not slept well some nights because of sudden onsets of night sweats. All of the symptoms he related to the stress of finishing college and looking for employment.

A chest x-ray ordered by his physician showed increased x-ray density in the right upper lung field, which exhibited the presence of several well-formed foci of high x-ray density. The results of a sputum culture confirmed the diagnosis of tuberculosis.

DELAYED-TYPE HYPERSENSITIVITY

Michael's immune system needs to stimulate his cell-mediated immune mechanisms to remove the *Mycobacterium tuberculosis* organism effectively. The term *cell-mediated immunity* encompasses the activities of both CD8 cytotoxic T cells and CD4 Th1 (helper T) cells. This second cell population is often referred to as Tdth cells. The target antigen for these two cell types and the nature of the resulting immune responses are different and are considered separately.

Biologic Role of DTH Reactions

Both Michael's PPD response and the immune response in his lung to the *M. tuberculosis*, which resulted in nodules of increased x-ray density, are examples of delayed-type hypersensitivity (DTH) reactions. These responses are mediated by cytokine products of the antigen-selected CD4 Th1 lymphocytes, or Tdth lymphocytes. These reactions are often considered to be inappropriate because they cause tissue damage (e.g., Michael's PPD response and lung granulomas), but that tissue damage is associated with critical protective immunity. Generally, in humoral responses, the antigen is transported to either the lymph nodes or spleen (IgG responses) or to the organized mucosal lymphoid tissues (IgA responses). In Michael's immune response to the mycobacteria, the organism is intracellular in the macrophages of the lungs, and therefore cannot be transported to the nodes. Other classic examples of DTH reactions include contact hypersensitivities, in which the stimulating agent is often a reactive chemical that can covalently modify cell-surface components of the contacted tissues and present the altered self-antigens to the immune system. Again, because of the tissue location, moving the antigen-modified cells to the nodes is not possible. The DTH response method induces a local inflammatory response and brings cells and other components of the immune system to the site of the tissue-localized antigen. In many respects, it can be thought of as similar to either the inflammatory functions of complement C3a or the IgE-mediated reactions, because all three send signals to the immune system, indicating a localized inflammatory reaction. The differences between immediate and delayed responses are outlined in Table 13-1.

TABLE 13-1 ▶

Delayed-Type versus Immediate-Type Hypersensitivity Responses

	Immediate Hypersensitivity	*Delayed Hypersensitivity*
Cell mediators	IgE and mast cells	CD4 Th1 cells
Chemical mediators	Histamine and synthesized mediators	Interferon-γ
Time required to observe reaction	Minutes	24–48 hours
Character of reaction	Edematous wheal and flair	Indurated swelling

Phases of the DTH Response

Role of CD8 T Cells in DTH Reactions.
The interferon-γ produced in DTH reactions brings many types of lymphocytes to the site of inflammation, including cytotoxic T cells (CTLs). These CTLs, like the other cells arriving at the inflammatory site, are activated and may play a role in the subsequent reaction.

Like all immunologic reactions, DTH reactions exhibit primary and secondary responses. The primary response in this case is often referred to as the sensitization phase. The visible manifestations of a primary DTH response are seldom evident because of an insufficient number of responding T cells. This primary response requires approximately 1–2 weeks to develop a sufficient number of antigen-specific Th1 cells. Fig. 13-1 outlines the events involved in the primary DTH response. This figure should be very familiar, because it reiterates the method of selecting CD4 lymphocytes.

The secondary response, or effector phase, of the DTH reactions results in a characteristic set of physical symptoms. On second exposure to antigen, there is a delayed (24–48 hours) swelling that is characterized by its indurated nature. Note that this is in contrast to immediate hypersensitivity reactions, in which the response is immediate and edematous. The DTH response usually peaks 2–3 days following the secondary exposure to antigen and then gradually diminishes in magnitude.

Fig. 13-2 outlines the events involved in the effector phase of DTH reactions. When antigen is encountered in a tissue, the resident macrophages process and present the antigen to CD4 Th1 cells. This response activates the selected Tdth cells in the area of the antigen insult, and the cell begins making and secreting interferon-γ (IFN-γ) in addition to other cytokines. In response to these cytokines, all nucleated cells in the area process and present antigen more rapidly. Resident macrophages are activated to increase their rate of phagocytosis and killing efficiency. The cytokine products of activated Tdth cells are also chemotactic, bringing into the area lymphocytes and monocytes that are responsible for the delayed indurated swelling.

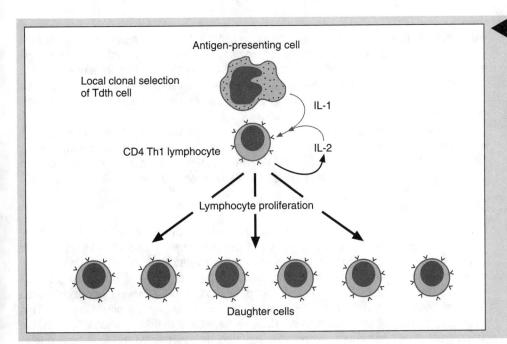

FIGURE 13-1
Primary or Sensitization Phase of the DTH Response. Localized antigen is presented by a resident macrophage to a CD4 Th1 (helper T) lymphocyte. With the cytokine help of interleukin-1 and -2 (IL-1, IL-2), the selected CD4 cell proliferates, producing daughter cells with identical antigen-binding specificity. The resulting daughter cells are now free to migrate to all other tissues and are capable of responding to class II major histocompatibility complex–presented antigen with the production of interferon-γ.

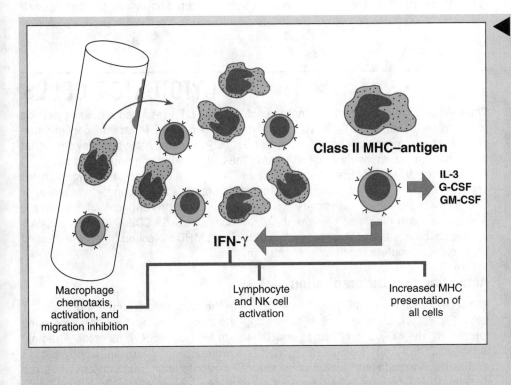

FIGURE 13-2
Effector Phase of the DTH Response. Following proliferation of the selected CD4 Th1 lymphocyte, subsequent exposure to the identical antigen results in the secretion of interferon-γ (IFN-γ). IFN-γ is chemotactic for macrophages and lymphocytes. The cytokine activates these cells and prevents them from leaving the area of the antigen. These activities are responsible for the delayed indurated swelling observed in DTH reactions. IFN-γ also increases the activity and expression of the major histocompatibility complex (MHC) on all nucleated cells in the area of the inflammation. In addition to IFN-γ, other cytokines are produced that promote eventual tissue repair and IL-3; granulocyte colony-stimulating factor (G-CSF), and granulocyte-macrophage colony-stimulating factor (GM-CSF) stimulate the bone marrow stem cell to increase production of lymphocytes, granulocytes, and monocytes. Chronic DTH stimulation leads the monocytes and macrophages to encapsulate the antigen source with epithelioid macrophages, lymphocytes, and fused multinucleate giant cells. This structure surrounding the antigen source is a granuloma. NK = natural killer.

Cytokine-mediated DTH Responses

Interleukin (IL)-1 and tumor necrosis factor (TNF), derived from the macrophage, stimulate the endothelial cells of the local capillaries to alter expression of their cell-adhesion molecules and allow inflammatory cells to leave the circulation and migrate to the inflammatory site. IFN-γ, derived from the selected CD4 Th1 lymphocyte, activates the infiltrating macrophages and other cells with cytotoxic activity. Moreover, the cytokines prevent the activated cells from leaving the inflammatory site. IFN-γ also increases the expression of the major histocompatibility complex (MHC) molecules on nonlymphoid cells. In this scenario, IFN-γ acts as a macrophage chemotactic factor (macrophage-activating factor) while it inhibits macrophages from leaving the inflammatory site (migration-inhibition factor). IFN-γ plays a key role in these DTH reactions. Individuals who are selectively missing the IFN-γ gene, not surprisingly, cannot mount successful DTH responses.

Another set of cytokines found in DTH reactions includes the hematopoietic growth and differentiation factors, such as IL-3 and granulocyte-macrophage colony-stimulating factor (GM-CSF). These factors stimulate the bone marrow stem cell population to proliferate and differentiate along the granulocyte-monocyte lineage.

Tissue Damage

Antigen is generally detectable by the DTH response with little damage to the local tissue. However, if there is persistent antigen stimulation, such as Michael's response to the *M. tuberculosis*, or if there is a significantly elevated number of Tdth-responding cells, the antigen source becomes encapsulated by the activated macrophages. The macrophages adhere to each other and take on an epithelial-like shape. Some cells even fuse into multinucleated giant cells, displacing and damaging the normal tissue. This structure, called a *granuloma*, can continue to form until there is a visable or palpable mass. In Michael, the area of increased x-ray density observed in the lungs was due to granuloma formation around sites of mycobacterial infection. Significant numbers of granulomas alter both the structure and function of affected tissue and can be responsible for a considerable amount of pathology.

CYTOTOXIC T CELLS

Cell-mediated immune reactions include not only the DTH response but also cytotoxic reactions mediated by the CD8 cytotoxic T lymphocyte (CTL). CTLs are the only immune cells able to survey the synthetic products of all host-nucleated cells, and they can either detect viral infection inside a cell or identify the cells making abnormal proteins.

Like the DTH response, the response of CTLs can be divided into two different phases: an initial primary response, or activation phase; and a secondary response, or effector phase, in which target cells expressing the stimulating antigens are specifically lysed. Since cell-mediated cytotoxicity is the domain of the CD8 T lymphocyte, this implies that the antigen for these reactions are class I MHC molecules holding processed viral products, mutated proteins, or tumor antigens.

Activation and Differentiation

The activation of the CD8 T lymphocyte duplicates the mechanisms for the activation of T cells (Fig. 13-3). Once selected by an appropriate class I MHC and antigen-expressing target cell, the CD8 T lymphocyte is activated to express an IL-2 receptor. Although activated CD8 T cells have been reported to synthesize IL-2, they apparently cannot synthesize it in sufficient amounts necessary for proliferation, and consequently, the selected CD8 T cell needs help from an appropriate IL-2–secreting CD4 helper T cell. The activated CD8 T lymphocyte that receives the IL-2 signal begins proliferating and differentiating either into an efficient antigen-specific CTL that can kill target cells or into a cytotoxic memory cell.

CTL Effector Phase

Following the initiation, proliferation, and differentiation of the selected CD8 T lymphocyte, there will be sufficient activated CTLs to seed all tissues. When one of these mature daughter cells encounters a target cell expressing the appropriate MHC–antigen complex, the two cells form a conjugate, and the CTLs release perforin monomers. Perforin monomer is a protein similar to the C9 component of complement. When it interacts with the target-cell membrane, it polymerizes and eventually creates pores in the target cell,

Role of CD4 Cells in CTL Responses.
As a result of CD8 T-cell–mediated cytotoxicity, components from the target cell are released into the interstitial space. These extracellular antigens can be processed and presented to CD4 lymphocytes. Consequently, the CD4 cells may also play multiple important roles in the CTL response. Not only can the CD4 cell provide the IL-2 that is necessary for CD8 proliferation, it can also initiate further inflammation by stimulating DTH reactions.

Costimulatory Signals.
Clonal selection of both CD4 and CD8 lymphocytes requires the interaction of several lymphocyte and antigen-presenting cell (APC) surface components, in addition to the MHC–antigen complex interaction with the T-cell receptor (TCR). Generally, APCs and all lymphocytes have these accessory molecules, and therefore, it is the antigen providing the critical component that permits clonal selection and the formation of the cell-surface macromolecular complex.

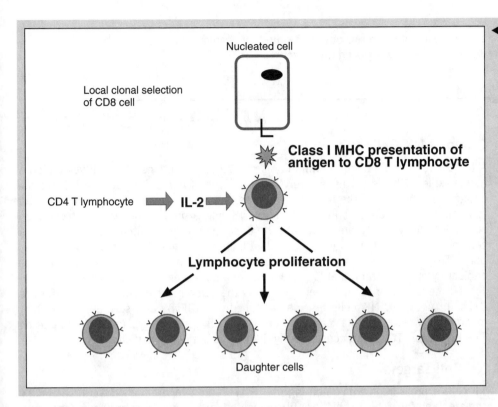

FIGURE 13-3
Activation of CD8 Cytotoxic T Cells. *CD8 lymphocytes are selected by processed antigen, presented by class I MHC molecules. The selected T lymphocyte expresses an IL-2 receptor, and on receiving IL-2 from a CD4 helper T lymphocyte, proliferates to daughter cells with an identical MHC-processed-antigen specificity. The resulting daughter cells can migrate to other tissues, and if the MHC-processed antigen that selected the parent CD8 cell is encountered, the daughter cells express a potent cytotoxic activity.*

much like the polymeric form of C9 (poly-C9) component of complement. Since one CTL is able to kill several target cells, the CTL either must have membrane components that resist the actions of perforin or must package and deliver the perforin monomers in such a way that the CTL is not exposed to the lytic agent. Fig. 13-4 illustrates the effector phase of the CTL response.

A second method that is called into action to destroy the target cell is the activation of the target cell's apoptotic mechanisms. The apoptosis activates nucleases that rapidly fragment nuclear material in the target cell. It is currently not clear what the relative

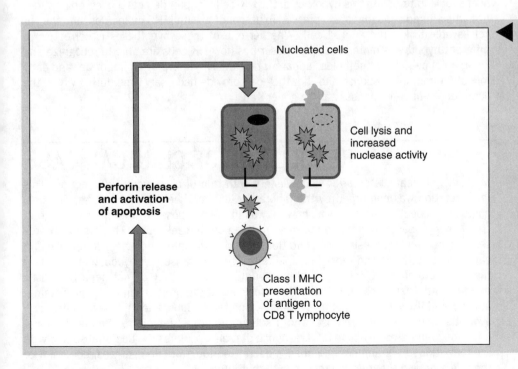

FIGURE 13-4
Effector Phase of the CD8 Cytotoxic T-Cell Response. *When one of the daughter cells derived from the selection of a CD8 lymphocyte encounters the appropriate MHC-processed-antigen complex, the cytotoxic T lymphocyte (CTL) releases perforins in the immediate location of the target cell and activates the apoptotic mechanisms in the target cell. The CTL leaves the target cell and is then ready to interact with another MHC-processed-antigen-presenting target. Perforins that were released at the target cell are lytic molecules, much like the C9 component of complement, and produce pores in the target cell membrane. The apoptotic mechanisms that are activated result in the digestion of the nuclear material in the target cell.*

contributions of these two different killing mechanisms are; however, both result in the death of the cell expressing the target antigen.

NATURAL KILLER CELLS

Origin of NK Cells

A third type of cell-mediated immunity is related to the actions of a cell type called a natural killer (NK) cell. This is a very different type of immunity, because it lacks the antigen dependency of the acquired immune responses. This type of immunity is an example of cell-mediated natural immunity. NK cells express some markers in common with T lymphocytes and are derived in the bone marrow as are other lymphocytes. NK cells are, however, clearly morphologically distinct from the other lymphocyte populations. They are large granular cells instead of small lymphoid cells, without a large nuclear:cytoplasmic ratio that is characteristic of both B and T lymphocytes.

NK cells appear to kill target cells using the same mechanisms described for the CTLs. In addition, NK cells are clearly sensitive to IFN-γ and several of the other inflammatory cytokines that can augment their killing efficiency. However, there is no T-cell receptor (TCR), and consequently there is no antigen specificity.

NK Cell Targets

NK cells express fragment combining site (Fc) receptors for antibody-coated target cells and are, therefore, able to kill the antibody-coated target through an antibody-dependent cell-mediated cytotoxic (ADCC) mechanism. However this ADCC mechanism does not explain NK-cell cytotoxic activity in the absence of antibody. The lack of antigen specificity presents a significant problem in understanding how NK cells function. There are at least two general hypotheses that address the issue, both of which are supported by current research. One hypothesis holds that when a cell's metabolism is altered (e.g., an infection) there are changes in the levels or nature of the class I MHC molecules. NK cells, then, may detect these alterations or may detect a decrease in the normal MHC density and kill the abnormal cell. A second hypothesis holds that cellular proteins are programmed to be expressed when the cell is experiencing abnormal conditions (e.g., heat shock proteins). In this hypothesis, the NK-cell receptor detects processed peptides from the altered cells that are expressed in association with MHC molecules, and the NK cell is able to kill the altered cell. Whether one of these hypotheses is correct, or a different hypothesis more accurately describes how NK cells are able to recognize and kill a target cell, it is nonetheless apparent that the NK cells play an important and early role in an immune response and that they can provide necessary time during which the acquired immune responses can be generated.

RESOLUTION OF CLINICAL CASE

Michael's clinical presentation is consistent with that of a tuberculosis infection. This interpretation was confirmed by the laboratory tests and cell culture results. The only confusing aspect of the case was how he was initially exposed to the infectious agent.

The mycobacteria infected the macrophages of Michael's lung. This organism possesses a cell wall that resists the conditions found in the interior of the macrophage and can successfully live and reproduce inside the cell. Because the mycobacteria contain their own protein-synthesizing machinery, unlike a virus, they do not need the host's protein-synthesizing machinery and, therefore, avoid the protein sampling, processing, and class I MHC expression of its synthesized proteins. Consequently, the organism can avoid the CD8 immune response, and it sets up a chronic infection. The chronic local infection stimulates an active DTH response that encapsulates the bacterial source with the formation of a granuloma. Michael's decreased lung function is the direct result of the infection and the immune response to that infection.

REVIEW QUESTIONS

Directions: For each of the following questions, choose the **one best** answer.

1. Which of the following cytokines is associated with the effector phase of a DTH reaction?
    (A) IL-1
    (B) IL-2
    (C) IL-8
    (D) IL-4 and IL-5
    (E) IFN-γ

2. Which of the following cells is associated with the sensitization phase of a DTH reaction?
    (A) CD4 Th1 lymphocyte
    (B) CD4 Th2 lymphocyte
    (C) CD8 T lymphocyte
    (D) Neutrophil
    (E) Mast cell

3. While playing in her backyard, Sally was stung on the arm by an insect. Over the course of the next 2 days, the tissue around the site of the bite turned red and was associated with an area of firm swelling. Which of the following is the most likely type of reaction taking place in Sally's arm?
    (A) IgE reaction
    (B) Activation of complement
    (C) CTL response
    (D) DTH reaction

4. While playing in his backyard, Billy was stung on the arm by an insect. Over the course of the next 2 minutes, the tissue around the site of the bite turned red and was associated with an edematous area of swelling. Which of the following is the most likely type of reaction taking place in Billy's arm?
    (A) IgE reaction
    (B) Activation of complement
    (C) CTL response
    (D) DTH reaction

5. A large area of indurated swelling was noted 48 hours after receiving an intradermal injection of PPD from a mycobacteria. A histologic section of the affected tissue would show elevated levels of which of the following cell types?
    (A) Lymphocytes
    (B) Macrophages
    (C) Neutrophils
    (D) Lymphocytes and macrophages
    (E) Macrophages and neutrophils

Note. Abbreviations used in the questions: DTH = delayed-type hypersensitivity; IL-1 = interleukin-1; IFN-γ = interferon-γ; IgE = immunoglobulin E; CTLs = cytotoxic T lymphocytes; PPD = purified protein derivative; MHC = major histocompatibility complex; APC = antigen-presenting cell; IL-4 = interleukin-4; NK = natural killer; TCR = T-cell receptor.

6. Long-term exposure of a tissue to *M. tuberculosis* results in damage to the tissue from which of the following mechanisms?

    (A) Antibody-dependent cell-mediated cytotoxicity

    (B) Release of eosinophil major basic protein

    (C) Cell death resulting from chronic CTL activity

    (D) Granuloma formation

    (E) Complement-mediated inflammation

7. Following clonal selection of a CD8 T lymphocyte, the necessary information to allow the selected cell to proliferate and differentiate is provided by which of the following activated cells?

    (A) The class I MHC APC

    (B) Clonal selection of the CD8 lymphocyte is sufficient, no additional help is necessary

    (C) IL-4 and IL-5 from a CD4 Th2 cell

    (D) IL-2 from a CD4 Th1 cell

8. The CTLs kill target cells using which of the following mechanisms?

    (A) Antibody and complement

    (B) Generation of reactive oxygen species

    (C) Recruitment and activation of monocytes

    (D) Liberation of pore-forming proteins and activation of apoptosis

9. Which of the following is a correct statement about NK cells?

    (A) NK cells are a type of T lymphocyte because they express the TCR.

    (B) NK cells are able to recognize specific antigens because they have a receptor for each individual antigen.

    (C) NK cells can be activated by IFN-γ.

    (D) NK cells use phagocytic mechanisms to kill target cells.

10. CD8 CTLs do not play a major role in the immune response against the intracellular *Mycobacterium tuberculosis* for which of the following reasons?

    (A) CD8 lymphocytes are not in the area of the infection.

    (B) The macrophage that is infected by *M. tuberculosis* displays cell-surface class II MHC molecules and not class I MHC molecules.

    (C) *M. tuberculosis* is not a dividing and growing organism.

    (D) *M. tuberculosis* does not use the host's protein-synthesizing machinery to synthesize proteins for bacterial growth.

ANSWERS AND EXPLANATIONS

1. **The answer is E.** During the primary, or sensitization, phase of DTH responses, IL-1 and IL-2 play a major role in the proliferation of the selected CD4 Th1 cells. However, when one of the daughter cells re-encounters the selecting antigen, IFN-γ plays the major role. The cytokine acts as a chemotactic factor for macrophages and lymphocytes and as a migration-inhibition factor that prevents inflammatory cells from leaving the site of inflammation. It is also an activating factor for multiple cell types, including macrophages and NK cells.

2. **The answer is A.** The cell responsible for DTH reactions is the CD4 Th1 lymphocyte. The CD4 Th2 lymphocyte, although also selected by class II MHC–presented antigen, functions to help selected B lymphocytes proliferate and switch isotypes. The CD8 T lymphocytes mediate antigen-dependent, cell-mediated cytotoxicity. Neutrophils depend on antibody to provide them with antigen specificity, while mast cells depend upon IgE or the anaphylatoxin components of complement.

3. **The answer is D.** A reaction that is delayed 24–48 hours and is characterized by an indurated swelling is a DTH reaction. One type of immunologic reaction that is sometimes confused with the DTH reaction is an Arthus reaction, or type III hypersensitivity reaction. This is a localized antigen–antibody reaction that is caused when antigen is deposited in the skin of a hyperimmunized host. This reaction is usually observed 4–8 hours after antigen administration, but, at low concentrations of either antigen or antibody, the reaction can be delayed even longer. The character of the Arthus reaction, however, differs. The antigen–antibody complex that is formed stimulates complement and phagocytes with the initial accumulation of neutrophils and is far more edematous and purulent.

4. **The answer is A.** This reaction is a classic definition of an immediate IgE reaction.

5. **The answer is D.** The PPD reaction is a classic example of a DTH reaction. Most DTH reactions involve an early transient increase of neutrophils because of the early macrophage stimulation; however, this initial response is overwhelmed by the influx of both lymphocytes and macrophages, which gives rise to the indurated swelling of the response.

6. **The answer is D.** Chronic DTH responses allow the lymphocytes and macrophages to encapsulate the source of the antigen and "wall off" the antigen source. The resulting granuloma displaces normal tissue and adversely affects its function.

7. **The answer is D.** Just as selected B cells need B-cell growth factors and differentiation factors from the CD4 cell population, the selected CD8 CTL needs T-cell growth factors to proliferate. In this case, the T-cell growth factor is IL-2.

8. **The answer is D.** The active CTL does not depend on other cells or factors to produce a cytotoxic effect. The CD8 cell contains packaged perforins that, when released, create pores in the target-cell membrane. In addition, nucleases are activated in the target cell.

9. **The answer is C.** NK cells are large granular lymphocytes, which express some cell-surface markers in common with other T lymphocytes, but not the TCR. NK cells recognize classes of cells that alter the expression of normal cell-surface components. Since the NK cell has a fragment combining site (Fc) receptor for antibody, it can also affect cell-mediated cytotoxicity in an antibody-dependent manner (antibody-dependent cell-mediated cytotoxicity). The activity of NK cells can be increased by IFN-γ and several other cytokines.

10. **The answer is D.** The class I MHC antigen-processing mechanism requires the material being synthesized to be marked with ubiquitin and processed by a proteasome in order to combine with the class I MHC molecule for presentation on the cell surface. The intracellular bacteria contain their own protein-synthesizing machinery, and consequently, bacterial antigens are not expressed. Viruses, on the other hand, use the host ribosomes and enzymes, and viral products are presented on the cell surface.

14 COMPLEMENT

INTRODUCTION OF CLINICAL CASE

Mrs. Jenkins, a 32-year-old African American, consulted her physician with complaints of malaise, lethargy, and body aches. During the interview with her physician, it became clear that her body aches and lethargy had been coming on for some time. The body aches seemed to involve both joints and muscles and could not be localized at any specific area of the body. Mrs. Jenkins was most concerned, however, about her recent weight loss and some irregular-shaped erythematous patches that had appeared on her face. She also had had a similar rash on her forearm 6 months ago, which resolved but left significant scarring and a loss of pigment.

Mrs. Jenkins's physical examination failed to identify much additional detail about her current problem other than there being no abnormalities associated with the joints where she indicated she was experiencing pain. There were, however, some ulcerations evident, but they were not localized. She also had some small cutaneous hemorrhages, and small ulcers were found on both her oral and genital mucosa.

In an attempt to identify the source of Mrs. Jenkins's problems, a battery of laboratory tests was ordered. One laboratory test identified her CH50 as extremely low. The CH50 test evaluated the total amount of complement components available to react with a standardized antigen–antibody complex. Mrs. Jenkins's CH50 data indicated either a problem producing the serum complement components or an abnormally high consumption of complement.

OVERVIEW

This chapter provides a detailed discussion of the initiation, amplification, and regulation of the complement system. The complement system has three distinct and critical biologic functions. These activities induce inflammation (anaphylaxis), opsonize parti-

Complement Functions
- *Anaphylaxis*
- *Opsonization*
- *Lysis*

cles for phagocytic removal, and lyse susceptible organisms. When considering the complement system in its entirety, the system can be visualized as consisting of three different phases: phase I is the activation phase of the response, phase II includes the amplification events, and phase III is the direct lysis of cells.

COMPLEMENT ACTIVATION

A **zymogen**, an inactive precursor to an active enzyme, is activated by proteolytically altering the peptide, which allows it to assume a different active conformation. In addition to the complement proteins, the clotting cascade and several of the digestive proteins are also zymogens.

The activation of the complement system is often considered the most difficult of the three phases to understand. This is undoubtedly because two different methods are employed to activate the system: the classic pathway and the alternate pathway. The end product of both complement activation pathways is the generation of the enzyme C3 convertase. This enzyme converts the serum zymogen C3 into two active components, C3a and C3b. Although there are amplification steps in the activation of complement, the enzyme C3 convertase can be viewed as the beginning of the phase II amplification events.

Classic Pathway Activation

Antibody is required to initiate the classic complement pathway (Fig. 14-1); therefore, complement activities are not available for immune protection until an antibody response has been generated.

FIGURE 14-1

Initiation of Classic Pathway. *Serum complement component C1q can bind to the adjacent Fc portions of two antibody molecules that have bound antigen. Binding to antibody induces a conformational change, which activates a protease activity in the C1r and C1s components of the C1 molecule. The protease is specific for serum complement component C4, cleaving it into a large C4b fragment and a small C4a fragment. The C4b fragment binds covalently to surfaces in the area where it was generated. The C4a peptide is soluble and has anaphylatoxin activity.*

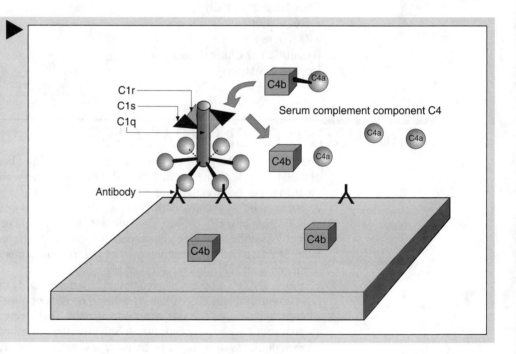

C2a
Warning: the fragments of complement component 2 are inconsistently named in textbooks. To simplify complement nomenclature, some define the large fragment of C2 that binds to C4b as C2b. However, some textbooks define the large fragment of C2 as C2a. This is the convention used here.

When an antigen–antibody complex is formed, the Fc portion of the antibody binds to a soluble set of serum proteins, the C1qrs components of complement. The binding of C1qrs to antibody induces a conformational change in the C1r and C1s components and activates in them a serine protease. The active C1qrs reacts with the complement component C4, a zymogen, cleaving a small peptide C4a from the zymogen and generating a C4b fragment that has binding affinity for membranes. As a result of this activity, the C1qrs protease enzymically produces several C4a and C4b products. The C4a peptide is an anaphylatoxin, while the C4b fragment forms covalent bonds with membranes and other surfaces.

The C1qrs enzyme also hydrolyzes complement component C2 into a small C2b peptide and a larger C2a fragment. The large C2a fragment combines with the surface-bound C4b to form C4bC2a, an intact C3 convertase enzyme capable of hydrolyzing serum complement component C3 into the C3a and C3b fragments.

Fig. 14-1 illustrates the C1q molecule interacting with the Fc portions of two antibody molecules. This is necessary to induce the conformational changes required to activate the C1r and C1s components of the C1 complex. Considering this requirement for two adjacent Fc fragments, immunoglobulin M (IgM) with its five connected Fc tails, not unexpectedly, is a very efficient activator of the complement system. Immunoglobulin G (IgG), on the other hand, requires an antigen concentration of sufficient density to allow two IgG molecules to be close enough to activate the complement system.

Alternate Pathway Activation

The second method by which complement can generate the critical C3 convertase enzyme is the alternate pathway, which does not require the presence of antibody. Consequently, if conditions are appropriate, the alternate complement pathway can activate inflammation (anaphylaxis), opsonize particles, and potentially lyse susceptible organisms without the delay required for antibody synthesis. This then is a rapid method of activating complement.

The alternate pathway depends on two competing reactions, both of which are also illustrated in Fig. 14-2. Complement component C3, the substrate for the enzyme C3 convertase, is continually being degraded at a relatively constant rate, generating the inflammatory C3a fragment and the opsonin C3b. Several enzymes, in addition to C3 convertase, can catalyze this proteolysis. These enzymes include proteases, which are normal cellular components, as well as some of the clotting enzymes. The generated amounts of these mediators are usually low. However, in the presence of either cellular damage or bleeding, the subsequent hydrolysis rate of C3 into the C3a and C3b fragments increases.

How would the complement system react with an IgG-coated antigen in which there was an insufficient antigen density to present two Fc tails close enough to interact with the same C1qrs complex?

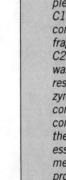

FIGURE 14-2
C3 Convertase Activity. In the classic complement pathway, the antibody-bound C1qrs protease acts on serum complement component C2, cleaving it into a large C2a fragment and a small C2b peptide. The C2a fragment associates with the C4b that was previously formed by the C1qrs. The resulting C4bC2a complex is a new enzyme called C3 convertase. The alternate complement pathway forms another C3 convertase from different components. In the alternate pathway, antibody is not necessary. The large C3b complement fragment is continually being generated by proteases. The resulting C3b is bound by either complement factor H or factor B. The factor H pathway leads to interaction with factor I and eventual inactivation. The factor B pathway, if stabilized, leads to processing by factor D and generates the C3 convertase, C3bBb. Both classic and alternate C3 convertase pathways have identical activities.

Alternate Pathway *C3 Convertase: C3bBb*
Classic Pathway *C3 Convertase: C4bC2a*

The C3b formed in hydrolysis can participate in one of two different reactions. In the first, C3b can bind to a serum factor called factor H to form the C3bH complex. This complex is a substrate for factor I, an enzyme that degrades the C3bH complex into inactive peptide. By following the factor H and factor I pathway, C3b is inactivated.

In the second reaction, the pathway available to C3b is to bind to serum factor B. This is a relatively unstable complex, which generally requires an appropriate surface to provide the necessary stability. The C3bB complex is a substrate for a serum protease called factor D, which cleaves a small peptide (Ba) from factor B, leaving the larger Bb fragment bound to C3b. This C3bBb complex is a second form of the enzyme C3 convertase. Initiation of both the classic and alternate pathways generates different forms of the same enzyme.

In summary, the alternate complement pathway consists of a set of two competitive pathways. One pathway leads to an active C3 convertase, while the other pathway results in inactive products. Under normal conditions, the pathway leading to inactivation predominates. However, if physiologic events lead to an increase in C3 production (e.g., bleeding) or if a surface is introduced that stabilizes the C3bBb complex (e.g., bacterial membrane or damage to a host membrane), then the C3 convertase pathway can successfully compete with the inactivation mechanisms, and a stable, active C3 convertase enzyme is formed, which can continue and can amplify complement reactions.

COMPLEMENT AMPLIFICATION

The C3 convertase generated in either the classic or alternate pathway catalyzes the proteolysis of complement component C3, generating two fragments. One fragment, C3a, is a small peptide, while the second and larger fragment, C3b, can covalently attach to surfaces. This reaction also illustrates the nature of amplification in zymogen reactions, showing how one C3 convertase enzyme can result in several hundred C3b molecules attached to a surface (Fig. 14-3).

FIGURE 14-3 ▶

Generation of C5 Convertase. *The enzyme C3 convertase, from either the classic or alternate pathway, rapidly increases the rate of C3b production. There are two fates for the large amount of C3b that is generated. Either it can bind covalently to the surfaces in the location where it was produced, or it can associate with the C3 convertase that was responsible for its generation. The surface-C3b is an opsonin for phagocytes. However, when C3b associates with the C3 convertase from either pathway, it changes the substrate specificity and converts the C3 convertase into a C5 convertase enzyme.*

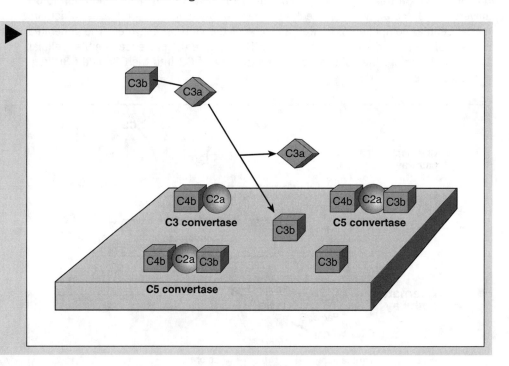

The products of the C3 convertase enzyme, **C3a** *and* **C3b,** *are responsible for anaphylatoxin and opsonization, respectively.*

Both products of the C3 convertase enzyme have critical roles in the biology of the complement system. Fragment C3a is an anaphylatoxin, which means that it binds to a specific receptor on the mast cell membrane and stimulates degranulation (see Chap. 2). Mast cell degranulation stimulates inflammation (anaphylaxis). The second C3 fragment, C3b, covalently binds to structures in the area where it was generated. Phagocytic cells that have receptors for the C3b component of complement can then efficiently phagocytize the C3b opsonized particles.

The C3b product of C3 convertase has an additional amplification function. This second function changes the substrate specificity of the C3 convertase (see Fig. 14-3). To accomplish this task, C3b interacts directly with the C3 convertase to form a new enzyme, C5 convertase. Similar activities are observed for the C3 convertase formed in both the classic and alternate complement pathways. In the classic pathway, the C4bC2a convertase is converted into a C4bC2aC3b trimolecular complex, which is a C5 convertase. In the alternate pathway, the C3bBb convertase is converted into a C3bBbC3b trimolecular complex, which also is a C5 convertase.

The C5 convertase continues the amplification of the complement response by cleaving the serum zymogen C5 into two fragments. This reaction generates a small C5a peptide, which has a very potent anaphylatoxin activity (Fig. 14-4). In addition, the larger C5b fragment can deposit over surfaces in the area where it was generated. In this sequence of steps, both the C3 convertase and the C5 convertase can eventually produce a large number of C5b molecules attached to the target membrane or surface. The C5b molecule begins the third or lytic phase of the complement system.

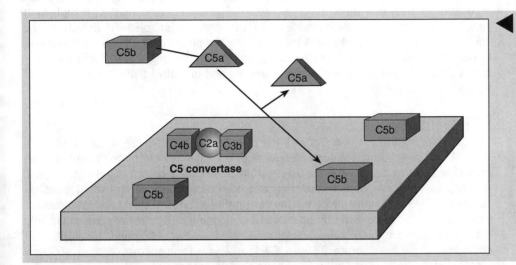

FIGURE 14-4

C5 Convertase Activity. *C5 convertase continues the amplification steps of the complement cascade. The large C5b fragment binds to surfaces, while the small C5a is, again, a soluble anaphylatoxin.*

LYSIS

The reactions involved in the lytic phase of complement (Fig. 14-5) begin with the C5b generated by C5 convertase during the amplification phase. C5b associates with complement factors C6, C7, and C8 to form a complex that converts the soluble C9 component of complement into a polymeric structure that inserts itself into the membrane, generating a pore. This polymeric C9 structure is the membrane attack complex (MAC) of complement. Unlike other complement activities, the generation of MAC does not depend on activation of zymogens; rather, the C5b organizes the C6, C7, and C8 components into a structure that induces conformational changes in the C9 component, promoting its polymerization and interaction with membrane lipids. With susceptible organisms, the generation of MAC results in cell lysis.

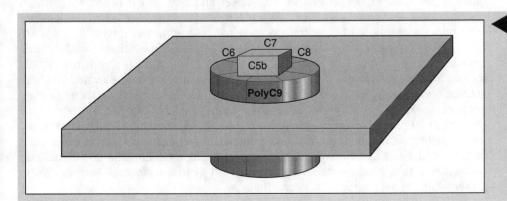

FIGURE 14-5

Lysis. *The C5b that is produced by C5 convertase is a nucleation point for the association of complement components C6, C7, and C8. Together, these fragments allow the C9 component of complement to aggregate into a membrane attack complex that eventually creates a pore in the susceptible target cell. Not all organisms are sensitive to complement-mediated lysis. PolyC9 = polymeric form of C9.*

COMPLEMENT ACTIVITY

Regulation

Complement has very potent activities and must be carefully regulated. Consequently, there are methods to shut down the activity of the system. Factor I, which has already been discussed in connection with the alternate complement pathway, is one of these regulators. In addition, there is an inhibitor of the C1qrs component of complement called *C1Inh*. This inhibitor dissociates the C1qrs complex and prevents its activity and activation of the classic pathway. A third inhibitor, found in host membranes but absent in bacterial membranes, is a protein called *decay accelerating factor (DAF)*. DAF promotes the breakdown of C3 convertase. There are also inhibitors that selectively prevent the formation of the MAC.

Measurement

Laboratory Measurement of the Complement System
CH50 *is a functional assay that measures the total amount of complement present and can be used to hemolyze antibody-coated erythrocytes.*

The laboratory data from Mrs. Jenkins's tests showed a significantly decreased CH50. The CH50 test is a functional measurement of the total amount of complement in an individual's serum that is available to lyse standard antibody-coated target erythrocytes. It measures total complement function but not the amounts of individual proteins. Decreased CH50 could result from a lack of synthesis, an increased level of consumption, or a defect in any one of the complement components. The clinical case should help distinguish between the possibilities. However, measurement of individual complement components, such as serum C3 and C4 levels, is an indispensable tool in clearly identifying the basis of any alteration in the complement system.

RESOLUTION OF CLINICAL CASE

In the context of her presentation, Mrs. Jenkins's low CH50 level suggested to the physician that she was chronically activating the complement system. Serum levels of both C3 and C4 were also low, which indicated that Mrs. Jenkins had been suffering from a chronic formation of antigen–antibody complexes, which were depositing in many of her organs and tissues. The rash, ulcers, and muscle and joint aches resulted from inflammatory activities associated with chronic complement activation by these complexes. There are, potentially, multiple sources of the antigen–antibody complex that can activate complement. Because of the insidious onset of Mrs. Jenkins's symptoms and because of the physical presentation, her physician initially elected to evaluate her serum for the presence of known autoantibodies. The autoantibody screen showed a much higher than expected level of antinuclear antibody, which is characteristic in systemic lupus erythematosus (SLE). As a result of unknown causes, Mrs. Jenkins has initiated an autoantibody response to nuclear antigens and, most probably, other unknown antigens. The resulting immune complexes deposited in her tissues and initiated immune complex or type III hypersensitivity reactions, which are primarily responsible for much of the pathology. Without obtaining test results showing elevated levels of antinuclear antibody, Mrs. Jenkins's condition, SLE, can be extremely difficult to diagnose because diagnosis depends both on the amount of autoantibody present and on the tissue distribution of the resulting immune complexes. To complicate diagnosis further, the circulating autoantibody is not always detected. Moreover, the complexes can deposit in different tissues in different patients, and in a single patient, the complexes may deposit in different tissues at different times. All of these variables lead to diverse presentations of patients with this condition.

REVIEW QUESTIONS

Directions: For each of the following questions, choose the **one best** answer.

1. Which of the following best describes the entire function of the complement system?
    (A) Anaphylaxis, opsonization, and cell-mediated lysis
    (B) Lysis of antibody-coated cells
    (C) Initiation of anaphylaxis
    (D) Anaphylaxis, opsonization, and lysis

2. Which of the following best describes the differences between the classic and alternate complement pathways?
    (A) The classic pathway results in the lysis of the target cell, which is not the case with the alternate pathway.
    (B) The alternate pathway requires antibody for initiation, and the classic pathway is antibody-independent.
    (C) The classic pathway is more active than the alternate pathway.
    (D) The alternate pathway requires either a stabilizing surface or an increase in the background rate of C3b production for activation, while the classic pathway requires adjacent antigen–antibody complexes.

3. Which of the following sets of complement fragments contains all of the biologic activities of the complement system?
    (A) C3a, C4a, and C5a
    (B) C3a, C3b, and the polymeric form of C9 (polyC9)
    (C) C3a, C5b-C6-C7-C8, and polyC9
    (D) C4b, C3b, and polyC9

4. An individual's finger was caught in a car door and, as a result, sustained significant tissue damage and internal bleeding without breaking the skin or infecting the wound with foreign materials. Which of the following is the most likely explanation for the resulting inflammation?
    (A) The inflammation must be the result of nonimmunologic mechanisms because there are no foreign antigens present.
    (B) The inflammation must be attributable to natural killer (NK) cells because they do not have a unique antigen receptor.
    (C) The inflammation is related to an increase in the amount of C4bC2a on the surface of the damaged tissue.
    (D) The inflammation is related to an increased constitutive production of C3b by clotting factors.

5. Clinical laboratory evaluation of a patient revealed significantly low CH50 and C3 levels but normal C4 levels. Which of the following is the most likely explanation for these data?
    (A) Activation of the classic complement pathway
    (B) Activation of the alternate complement pathway
    (C) A genetic deficiency in the classic pathway
    (D) A genetic deficiency in the alternate pathway

6. Clinical laboratory evaluation of a patient revealed significantly low CH50, C3, and C4 levels. Which of the following is the most likely explanation for these data?

   (A) Activation of the classic complement pathway

   (B) Activation of the alternate complement pathway

   (C) A genetic deficiency in the classic pathway

   (D) A genetic deficiency in the alternate pathway

7. Clinical laboratory evaluation of a patient revealed a significantly low CH50 and normal C3 and C4 levels. Which of the following is the most likely explanation for these data?

   (A) Activation of the classic complement pathway

   (B) Activation of the alternate complement pathway

   (C) The above data indicate a possible deficiency in the complement system.

   (D) The above data are not possible because a low CH50 must be associated with a low C3 level.

8. An Rh-negative mother had a significant anti-Rh response following the birth of her Rh-positive child. The maternal immunoglobulin G (IgG) coated the child's erythrocytes with antibody. However, the serum complement CH50 was not significantly decreased in the presence of severe hemolytic disease of the newborn. Which of the following best explains these data?

   (A) Complement is being fixed by the alternate pathway, which is not measured by the CH50 test.

   (B) Antibodies are directly cytotoxic to erythrocytes.

   (C) The Rh antigens must have a relatively low density on the cell surface and cannot activate C1qrs.

   (D) Erythrocytes are insensitive to the polyC9 component of complement and do not lyse; therefore, the CH50 will be normal.

ANSWERS AND EXPLANATIONS

1. **The answer is D.** The complement system is very versatile and plays multiple roles in the immune response. The three major functions of the system are initiating inflammation, opsonizing cells, and direct lysing of some target cells. The lytic mechanisms do not require additional cell-mediated help.

2. **The answer is D.** Although constructed differently, the enzyme C3 convertase is a common element in both pathways. The differences in the two pathways reside only in the method used to initiate the construction of C3 convertase. The classic pathway is totally dependent on antibody, while the alternate pathway requires a stabilizing surface and an increase in the normal rate of C3b production.

3. **The answer is B.** The enzyme C3 convertase is critical in that it can produce both the anaphylatoxin C3a and the opsonin C3b. The other small fragments of the complement system also have anaphylatoxin activity. The remaining function of the complement system, cell lysis, depends on the formation of the polyC9.

4. **The answer is D.** In the presence of increased clotting enzymes or an alteration to the surface of the damaged cells, the alternate pathway of complement activation is increased, and the inflammatory mechanisms are stimulated by antigen-independent mechanisms.

5. **The answer is B.** The low CH50 and C3 levels indicate either that the complement system is inactive or that the complement components have been consumed. The normal C4 value rules out the activation of complement via the classic pathway.

6. **The answer is A.** Because C4 and C3 are both being consumed, the classic pathway has been activated. The extent of the alternate pathway's contribution to the C3 consumption is unknown.

7. **The answer is C.** Because the C3 levels are normal and because both the classic and alternate pathways use C3, the results suggest that complement is not being activated or consumed. In this case, one is left with the belief that the low CH50 may result from either elevated levels of complement inhibitors or a complement deficiency.

8. **The answer is C.** The maternal response to the Rh antigen is of the IgG class. If the antigen is of insufficient density, the classic complement pathway is not initiated. In this case, the hemolysis is due to phagocytosis and not complement-mediated lysis.

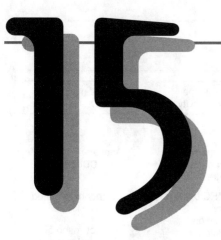

IMMUNOLOGIC TISSUE DAMAGE

INTRODUCTION OF CLINICAL CASE

Jimmy Otis, an 8-year-old, was rushed to the emergency room by his parents when they noticed that the color of Jimmy's urine was dark "like cola." Jimmy's medical history was significant for a sore throat 2 weeks previously that went untreated. The infection, however, was self-limiting and eventually resolved. The parents related that Jimmy had never had a similar incident of dark urine, and there was no family history of a similar problem. Analysis showed blood in the urine. Moreover, blood levels of urea nitrogen and creatinine confirmed kidney damage. High serum levels of antibody for the streptococcal antigens suggested that Jimmy's recent sore throat was caused by that organism.

TISSUE DAMAGE ASSOCIATED WITH IMMUNOLOGIC REACTIONS

Fig. 15-1 schematically summarizes the array of immunologic reactions that can be used to remove antigen. How these mechanisms are initiated and how they work to remove antigen has been one of the central foci of this study of the basic principles of immunology. Each of the mechanisms that can remove antigen is coupled to extremely potent activities that are capable of killing foreign cells. These cytotoxic activities are directed at the foreign cell by specific antibody and by the specificity of the T-cell receptor. Nevertheless, in the presence of activated phagocytes and other cytotoxic cells, in addition to the inflammatory mediators, there is modification and damage to normal tissues. The reactions that damage normal tissues at a level that can be detected clinically are termed *hypersensitivity reactions*. Hypersensitivity reactions are classified in four distinct types, which relate both to the immunologic effector mechanisms previously discussed and to the nature of the immune response that elicits the damage (Table 15-1). Jimmy's kidney problem, a direct result of his previous strep throat, provides an excellent example of how tissue damage associated with a successful immunologic reaction can lead to serious pathology.

FIGURE 15-1

Effector Mechanisms of the Immune System. *Summarized in this figure is the array of immunologic mechanisms that can be focused on antigen either to kill a viable cell or remove the remaining cellular debris. Many of the mechanisms involve extremely toxic molecules. Activated neutrophils and other phagocytes contain hydrolytic enzymes, acids, and active-oxygen species that can damage not only the target cell but also host cells. Complement activation initially induces tissue edema and inflammation, which can alter structure. The complement system also marks all cells in the area of activation with C3b, which, in turn, marks them for removal by the phagocytic system. IgE anaphylaxis immediately induces tissue edema but also recruits eosinophils, which contain a toxic basic protein in their granules. The cell-mediated immunologic mechanisms induce structural alterations in tissues, resulting from delayed-type hypersensitivity reactions, and can even result in the formation of granulomas. Cytotoxic T cells have a direct cytotoxic effect on any cell expressing a major histocompatibility complex (MHC)–target antigen complex. ADCC = antibody-dependent cell-mediated cytotoxicity; BcR = B-cell receptor for antigen.*

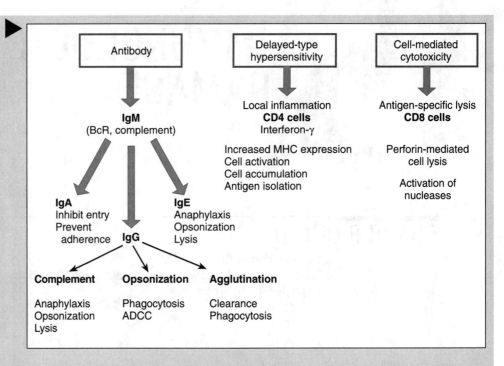

TABLE 15-1

Hypersensitivity Reactions

Type	Name	Mechanism
I	Immediate	IgE-mediated
II	Autoantibody	Complement and ADCC
III	Immune complex	Complement and ADCC
IV	Cell-mediated	
	DTH	CD4 T cells
	CTL	CD8 T cells

Note. ADCC = antibody-dependent cell-mediated cytotoxicity; DTH = delayed-type hypersensitivity; CTL = cytotoxic T lymphocyte.

HYPERSENSITIVITY REACTIONS

Type I

The term type I, or immediate, hypersensitivity reactions refer to the immunoglobulin E (IgE)–mediated allergic and anaphylactic reactions. The mechanisms initiating these reactions as well as the toxic mechanisms were covered in Chap. 11. The reactions are characterized by an immediate (within minutes) edematous response (wheal and flair), followed by a slower indurated swelling. These two responses, as discussed earlier, result from the preformed and synthesized mediators of anaphylaxis. In both the immediate and delayed responses, there can be significant tissue damage.

Symptoms associated with the immediate response vary in different species, but generally, in less than a minute, blood pressure decreases, and the bronchioles and the intestinal and bladder muscles contract. All this is brought on by the massive tissue edema that is secondary to release of the preformed vasoactive amines. Similar mechanisms take place in both the localized and systemic reactions, the major difference being the amount and the location of the antigen. During this initial rapid reaction, tissue damage results from edema and the activities of the vasoactive amines.

During the slow reaction of anaphylaxis, tissue damage is secondary to the release of the cytokines and lipid mediators, as well as to the activities of the infiltrating inflammatory cells. Chronic stimulation of IgE reactions, such as that seen in asthma, results in additional events leading to tissue damage. One type of cell arriving later in the IgE response is the eosinophil. These cells contain within their granules a basic protein that has potent cytotoxic activity. Moreover, much of the tissue damage is the result of the cell-growth-and-repair cytokines liberated by the activated monocytes. Cytokines such as transforming growth factor (TGF), platelet-derived growth factor (PDGF), and fibroblast growth factor (FGF) lead to the development of scar tissue, which replaces cells having an important functional activity in the inflamed tissue.

Type II

Type II hypersensitivity reactions are antibody-mediated reactions, which include autoantibodies directed to self-tissues. These reactions usually manifest within hours of the antigen exposure. They are characterized by antibody-identifying cells, which are marked for destruction by phagocyte-mediated lysis (antibody-dependent cell-mediated [ADCC] cytotoxicity) or by antibody- and complement-induced inflammation.

It is important to point out that type II reactions are not limited to autoimmune responses. Some therapeutic compounds are alkylating or acylating agents, which can chemically modify tissue components and induce a response to a modified self-structure. When the drug is administered a second time, there is an immune response to drug-modified tissues. The immune response can take several forms: if the immune response generated is IgE in nature, then subsequent exposure to the agent results in a type I hypersensitivity reaction. However, if the response is of the IgG isotype, then a type II hypersensitivity reaction results. Type II hypersensitivity reactions can also be observed whenever there is a passive transfer of a tissue-specific antibody, such as the hemolytic disease of the newborn that results from the passive transfer of maternal antibody to an Rh-positive fetus. Fig. 15-2 summarizes the immunologic mechanisms that damage healthy tissue in type II reactions.

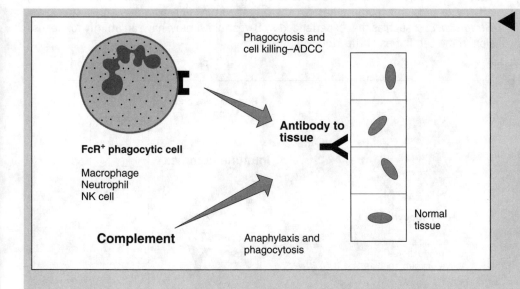

◀ **FIGURE 15-2**

Type II Hypersensitivity Reactions. Antibody-mediated reactions can damage host tissues using two different mechanisms. One method of damaging tissue relies on antibody to mark a tissue for destruction by Fc receptor (FcR)–bearing phagocytic cells. The phagocytic cell cannot differentiate between self- and nonself-components. Consequently, any cell marked with antibody will be phagocytosed and destroyed by the lysosomal enzymes, acid, and active-oxygen species of the phagocyte. The second method of damaging tissue is through the activation of complement via the classic pathway. In this case, complement induces inflammation, the physical alteration of tissue resulting from edema and the activation of phagocytes. Note that the mechanisms are identical to the mechanism used to remove any foreign antigen. NK = natural killer; ADCC = antibody-dependent cell-mediated cytotoxicity.

Type III

The third classification of hypersensitivity reaction derives from the tissue damage that is secondary to the deposition of immune complexes. Therefore, type III hypersensitivity reactions are detected following a successful immune response. Fig. 15-3 uses the familiar antigen clearance curve to follow the course of an immune response. Indicated in this figure is the period of time during which antigen–antibody complexes can be detected. It is during this period, when an individual is recovering from his or her antigen exposure, that type III hypersensitivity reaction can be observed.

FIGURE 15-3 ▶

Immune Complex Kinetics. Following a successful immune response, viable organisms are killed, and the resulting antigen fragments are removed by the reticuloendothelial system. The period during which immune complexes are at their highest concentration coincides with the immune elimination phase of antigen metabolism. Immune complexes can activate both phagocytes and complement, resulting in the host response to the immune complex–induced inflammation. The reaction to immune complexes is called serum sickness, and it is usually observed following administration of an antigenic therapeutic agent or an incompatible transfusion. Immune complex disease can also be observed following the successful response to a rapidly growing bacterium or virus.

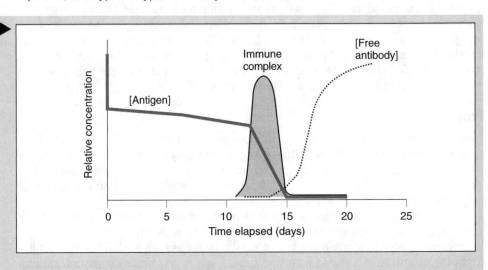

Depending on the size and nature of the complex, immune complexes that are normally cleared by the reticuloendothelial system can be deposited in capillaries. These complexes then present aggregations of antibody and antigen and use all of the methods normally employed by antibody to eliminate antigen (Fig. 15-4). As a result, the immune complex is removed, and any normal tissue in the location of the complex is also damaged by the inflammatory reaction. Immune complexes often exhibit tropism for tissues. The tropism appears to depend on the size of the complex, as well as on any affinity or cross-reactivity it has for the target tissue. For example, some species of *Streptococcus*, such as that experienced by 8-year-old Jimmy, have an affinity for deposition in the capillaries of the kidney glomerulus.

FIGURE 15-4 ▶

Type III Hypersensitivity Reactions. The complexes that are generated in an immunologic reaction can lodge in capillaries in various organs. Some of the more common sites are the skin, kidney, and joints. Immune complexes stimulate both phagocytes and complement, as described for type II hypersensitivity reactions. Activation of these systems results in tissue damage. The mechanisms of tissue damage for type II and type III hypersensitivity reactions are identical. However, the therapeutic intervention may differ significantly, depending on the source of the autoantibody that causes the type II reactions.

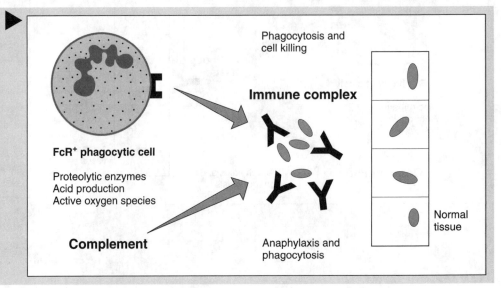

Type IV

Type IV hypersensitivity reactions are cell-mediated and include the reactions of cytotoxic CD8 T lymphocytes, as well as the delayed-type hypersensitivity (DTH) reactions mediated by the CD4 Th1 cells. Two totally different immunologic mechanisms are responsible for type IV hypersensitivity reactions.

The tissue damage that results from the CD8 cell follows directly from the killing of virus-infected cells by the cytotoxic T lymphocyte (CTL). It is easy to conceive how a tissue infected by a virus that does not cause major damage can be damaged and potentially rendered nonfunctional by the immune response to the virus. In some situations, the immune response to the virus is responsible for significantly more damage to the organ than the virus infection itself.

Type IV cell-mediated hypersensitivity reactions also include tissue damage caused by DTH responses. In this case, the tissue damage is secondary to the activities of interferon-γ (IFN-γ), and results from the activation of the local cells and the infiltration and subsequent activation of the monocytes and lymphocytes. These type IV hypersensitivity reactions employ the normal mechanisms used in the removal of antigen. Tissue damage is associated with the response to and removal of all antigens. However, only when the antigen load is excessive, or when there is chronic stimulation by the antigen, is the pathology associated with the immune reaction observed.

There is an additional, clearly recognized form of tissue damage associated with chronic DTH reactions—the formation of granulomas. When antigen chronically stimulates the immune system, DTH reactions recruit lymphocytes and monocytes to the location of the chronic stimulation and encapsulate the antigen source. The monocytes are activated; several take on a more epithelial shape; and some of the cells even fuse, creating multinucleate giant cells. This granuloma formation continues to grow, surrounding the antigen source, disrupting the architecture of the normal tissue, and altering its function.

RESOLUTION OF CLINICAL CASE

Jimmy had an untreated sore throat that eventually resolved. During the 2 weeks following the onset of the streptococcal infection, Jimmy's immune system mounted a response and generated a significant level of antibody to the organism (poststreptococcal glomerulonephritis). Immunologic mechanisms rapidly killed the organism and liberated soluble antigens that reacted with the antibodies to the organism. The time course of this response can be seen in Fig. 15-3. Immune complexes from the strain of the streptococcal organism that infected Jimmy have a tropism for the kidney glomerulus. The complexes lodge in the glomerulus and activate the complement system. In addition, complexes activate phagocytes, which then attempt to engulf the complexes. In the process, the phagocytes liberate their lysosomal contents, as well as the toxic active-oxygen species generated by stimulated phagocytes. Complement anaphylaxis opsonization and activated phagocytes contributed to the kidney damage in Jimmy.

REVIEW QUESTIONS

Directions: For each of the following questions, choose the **one best** answer.

1. Which of the following immune effector functions is responsible, in part, for the damage caused by type I hypersensitivity reactions?
   (A) Complement
   (B) Phagocytosis of tissue components
   (C) Tissue responses to interferon-γ
   (D) Eosinophil granule contents

2. Which of the following immune effector functions is responsible, in part, for the damage caused by type II hypersensitivity reactions?
   (A) Complement
   (B) Tissue responses to interferon-γ
   (C) Cytotoxic T lymphocyte–mediated killing of cells
   (D) Eosinophil granule contents

Directions: The group of questions below consists of lettered choices followed by several numbered items. For each numbered item, select the appropriate lettered option with which it is most closely associated. Each lettered option may be used once, more than once, or not at all.

Questions 3–10
For each clinical situation listed below, select the reaction that is most likely to be associated with it.
   (A) Type I hypersensitivity reaction
   (B) Type II hypersensitivity reaction
   (C) Type III hypersensitivity reaction
   (D) Type IV hypersensitivity reaction

3. Hemolytic disease of the newborn results when passively transferred antibody from the mother reacts with the neonate's erythrocytes.

4. Tissue damage is associated with chronic allergen exposure to the lung.

5. In myasthenia gravis, antibodies bind to the acetylcholine receptor and prevent the binding of acetylcholine. The resulting inability of the muscle to respond is functional tissue damage.

6. In rheumatoid arthritis, rheumatoid factor (antibody to the immunoglobulin molecule)–antigen complexes deposit in the joints, resulting in an inflammatory reaction.

7. Poststreptococcal glomerulonephritis appeared 2 weeks after a streptococcal infection.

8. Granuloma formation is associated with the immune response to *Mycobacterium tuberculosis.*

9. Eight hours following an injection of penicillin, a patient developed a purulent lesion at the injection site.

10. Contact dermatitis is observed in response to nickel-containing jewelry.

ANSWERS AND EXPLANATIONS

1. **The answer is D.** Immediate damage in a type I hypersensitivity reaction is caused by the tissue response to histamine. The lipid mediators of the anaphylactic reaction continue the tissue damage, as does the response to the cytokines released from the degranulated mast cells. Eosinophils arrive late in the course of immunoglobulin E (IgE)–mediated reactions. These cells contain a basic protein in their granules, which has potent cytotoxic activity.

2. **The answer is A.** There are two mechanisms of tissue damage in type II hypersensitivity reactions. These methods depend either on the activation of complement or on antibody-dependent cell-mediated cytotoxicity, in which Fc receptor–positive phagocytes and natural killer cells are directed to antibody-coated target cells.

3–10. **The answers are: 3-B, 4-A, 5-B, 6-C, 7-C, 8-D, 9-C, 10-D.** Although the hemolytic antibody is passively acquired and not produced by the child, it binds to the Rh antigens on the child's erythrocytes. Therefore, this is an antibody to a tissue, and it is a type II hypersensitivity reaction.

Allergic reactions are immediate hypersensitivity reactions, also called type I hypersensitivity reactions.

In this form of type II hypersensitivity reaction, not only can antibody induce complement activity and stimulate phagocytes, but it can also cause damage by blocking the function of a normal receptor. In some situations, such as Graves disease in which there is autoantibody to the thyroid-stimulating hormone receptor, the antibody actually mimics thyroid-stimulating hormone (TSH) and causes tissue damage by chronically stimulating the gland. This type of autoantibody-mediated tissue damage is sometimes referred to as a type V, or stimulatory, hypersensitivity reaction.

In rheumatoid arthritis, the immune complexes lodge in the joints and other tissues. This then is a type III, or immune complex, hypersensitivity reaction.

In addition to autoimmunity to a soluble protein causing a type III reaction, a large dose of a soluble antigen from either an infectious organism or an antigenic therapeutic agent also results in immune complexes that lodge in tissues and stimulate inflammatory tissue damage.

Granuloma formation is the result of chronic delayed-type hypersensitivity reactions and is therefore a form of type IV hypersensitivity reaction.

The timing of the reaction rules out an immediate hypersensitivity reaction, and the purulent nature of the lesion identifies it as an edematous infiltrate, containing neutrophils. The most likely explanation is that the individual who received the penicillin injection had a pre-existing immunoglobulin G (IgG) reaction to the drug; thus, the reaction is immune complex in nature.

Contact dermatitis reactions are usually delayed-type hypersensitivity reactions. In this case, the reactive metal is able to modify normal tissue components. This is a secondary response, indicating previous exposure to the metal-modified self-components.

16 MEASUREMENT OF IMMUNE RESPONSES

INTRODUCTION OF CLINICAL CASE

Karen Romero, 25 years old, went to see her physician, complaining of being tired and run-down. Because of her lack of energy, she had given up her daily exercise program, a routine that she had maintained for several years. Until a year ago, she was very active and considered herself to be in excellent physical condition. However, in the last year, she experienced several protracted colds and had three yeast infections, never previously a problem. During Karen's physical examination, the physician noted that several of her lymph nodes were enlarged, yet no current infection was evident. The physician then had the task of evaluating Karen's immune system to see if abnormalities in its response were the source of her problems.

HUMORAL IMMUNITY

Analysis of antibody levels is routinely performed in the clinical chemistry laboratory. The tests can provide a tremendous amount of information, not only about an individual's past experience with infectious disease, but also about the general health and functioning of the immune system itself. All serologic reactions depend on the following reaction:

$$\text{Antigen} + \text{antibody} \leftrightarrow \text{antigen–antibody complex}$$

Precipitation and Agglutination Reactions

The above reaction is detected by following the formation of the antigen–antibody complex. If the reactants are soluble and the complex precipitates, it is called a *precipitation reaction*. On the other hand, if the antigen is an insoluble particle, antibody will aggregate, or agglutinate, the particles. *Agglutination reactions* are classified by the type of insoluble particle (Table 16-1).

TABLE 16-1 ▶

Agglutination Reactions

Type	Insoluble Particle
Hemagglutination	Red blood cells
Bacterial agglutination	Bacteria
Passive agglutination	Soluble antigen coupled to an insoluble particle (usually blood cells or latex particles) to test for soluble antibody or antigen

Both agglutination reactions and precipitation reactions are extremely versatile. Not only can soluble antigens be detected by methods of passive agglutination, but analyses can be set up to evaluate the ability of a soluble particle to inhibit a standardized agglutination reaction (Fig. 16-1).

FIGURE 16-1 ▶

Precipitation Reactions. *When soluble antigen and antibody are mixed in the proper proportions, they form a large insoluble complex that can be visibly detected as a precipitate. If the antigen is an insoluble particle, or if a soluble antigen is coupled to an insoluble particle, the resulting reaction is called an agglutination reaction. The reaction can be easily measured by isolating the precipitate or agglutinate and determining how much of the material is present. If the amounts necessary to obtain a maximum precipitation of both antigen and antibody are mixed with additional soluble antigen, then the additional antigen interferes with the precipitation, producing smaller soluble complexes. Both the precipitation reaction and the inhibition of a precipitation reaction can be used to quantitate concentrations of either antigen or antibody.*

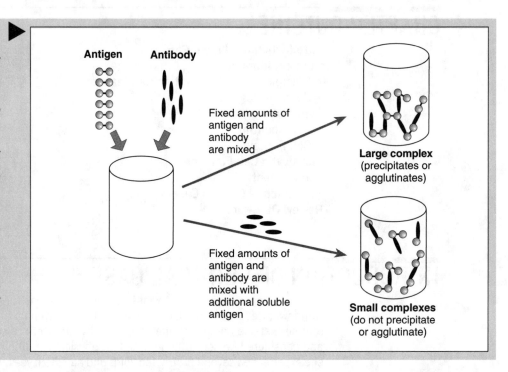

Coombs' Test
One common application of agglutination reactions is the detection of antibodies and autoantibodies to human erythrocyte antigens. In this test, erythrocytes coated with human antibody are mixed with a reagent containing antibodies to the human antibody (i.e., antihuman immunoglobulin). If the initial antibody density on the erythrocyte is sufficient, the addition of the antihuman immunoglobulin reagent will cause the erythrocytes to agglutinate. This test, called a direct antiglobulin test (AGT) or direct Coombs' test, is used extensively in blood typing and investigating autoimmune hemolytic anemia. An indirect form of the test can be used to measure soluble serum antibody.

The precipitation and agglutination assays provide flexible and useful methods for quantitating either antibody or antigen concentrations. To evaluate the antibody response to an infectious organism, a fixed amount of antigen from the suspected infectious agent is placed in test tubes containing dilutions of serum from an infected individual. After a suitable reaction period, chemical methods are used to measure the amount of precipitation or agglutination. The results of the analysis resemble the curve shown in Fig. 16-2. This precipitation curve shows three different zones for the reaction. In one zone, the antigen present exceeds the added antibody, and the amount of precipitate or aggregate is less than maximum. In the zone where there is an equivalence of antibody and antigen, one finds a maximum amount of either precipitate or agglutinate. In the third zone, antibody is in excess, and the amount of detected precipitate or agglutinate is again suboptimal. To evaluate the relative antibody levels in two different individuals, this test is performed on serum from each. If an individual has a high concentration of antibody in his or her serum, the serum must be diluted significantly more to reach the point of maximum precipitation than it would if the serum had a low antibody concentration (Fig. 16-3). In this test, serial dilutions from two different individuals are mixed with a constant amount of antigen, and the amount of precipitate is determined by either chemical or physical methods. The maximum amount that serum can be diluted and still produce a reaction is referred to as the *antibody titer*. The titer is the number that is reported to the physician when he or she requests serologic analyses of specific antibody levels.

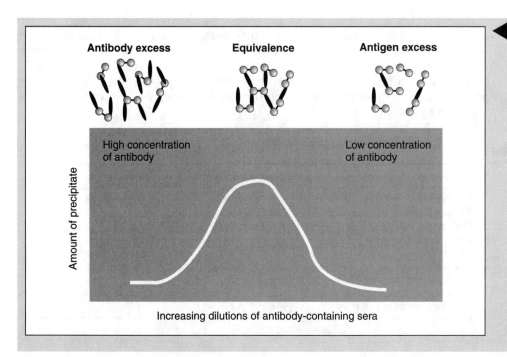

Figure 16-2

Precipitation Curve. When serum containing antibody is mixed with antigen, it is not always possible to know if the relative concentrations of antigen and antibody are at the proper proportions to obtain a maximum precipitate or agglutinate. To address this difficulty, a constant amount of antigen is mixed with serial dilutions of each antibody-containing serum. In this experiment, the amount of precipitate formed will vary. There are three broad zones to this precipitation curve: (1) the zone in which the amount of antibody exceeds that of antigen, (2) the zone of equivalence, and (3) the zone in which the amount of antigen exceeds that of antibody. The largest antigen–antibody complex occurs at the zone of equivalence, and consequently, the amount of precipitate is greatest in this zone. In each of the other two zones, the antigen–antibody complexes are smaller and do not precipitate as completely.

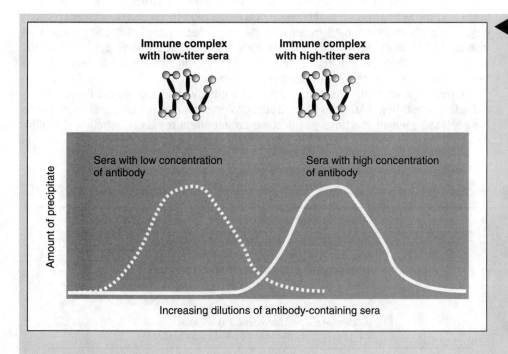

Figure 16-3

High-Titer versus Low-Titer Antisera. This figure compares the precipitation curves for two different serum samples. One sample contains a low concentration of antibody; the other sample contains a high concentration of antibody. Serial dilutions of both are mixed with a constant amount of antigen, and the amount of antigen–antibody precipitate is measured. Both the antigen–antibody complex and the ratio of antigen to antibody necessary to obtain a maximum amount of the immune complex are identical for each serum sample. Consequently, to obtain a maximum amount of precipitate, the serum sample containing more antibody must be diluted further than the serum sample with a low concentration of antibody. The amount that the serum must be diluted to obtain a defined level of precipitate is called the antibody titer. This is the number that clinical laboratories report to describe antibody concentration. High titers indicate high antibody concentrations; low titers indicate low antibody concentrations.

Coupled Reactions

Although the precipitation and agglutination assays can provide the data needed by a physician, these reactions are cumbersome, being slow and of insufficient sensitivity for many applications. Consequently, several modifications to these assays are in current use. Some modifications continue to detect antigen–antibody reactions by the precipitation reaction, except that the reaction is carried out in a gel matrix instead of in solution. Other modifications, however, couple the antigen–antibody reaction to techniques that allow the resulting complex to be detected using radiochemical, enzyme, or fluorescent techniques. These chemical modifications allow the clinical chemist to detect exceedingly low concentrations of either antigen or antibody. All of the techniques depend on the basic antigen–antibody reaction, but they differ in the methods of detecting the antigen–antibody complex or in the methods of separating complexes from free antigen and antibody, or both. Some frequently used methods are outlined in Table 16-2. Methods vary in sensitivity, from those that can detect mg/mL levels of antigen or antibody to sensitivities that can detect trace levels of hormones and even molecules produced by a single cell.

TABLE 16-2 ▶
Selected Methods for Measuring Antigen–Antibody Reactions

Name	Separation Method	Detection
Precipitation in solution	Centrifugation	Protein analysis
Radial diffusion	Diffusion in gel	Visual
Ouchterlony (double diffusion)	Diffusion in gel	Visual
Immunoelectrophoresis	Diffusion in gel	Visual
Nephelometry	None required	Light scattering
Coupled assays	Multiple methods	Dependent upon the agent
Radioimmunoassay (RIA)		
Enzyme immunoassay (EIA)		
Fluoroimmunoassay (FIA)		

The applications of antigen–antibody reactions also extend to microscopic investigations of tissues, in which antibody specifically binds to structures on a histologic section. If the antibody used in this protocol is either modified with a fluorescent reagent (e.g., fluorescein) or coupled to an enzyme (e.g., peroxidase) that can produce an insoluble product, then the coupled antibody reagent binds to and outlines specific antigenic structures on the tissue section. This immunohistochemical technique is termed immunofluorescent, or immunoenzyme, microscopy.

A modification of the immunofluorescent antibody technique called fluorescence-activated cell sorting (FACS), in which a suspension of fluorescent antibody-coated cells are analyzed one cell at a time, has become an important research and clinical tool for cell counting and analysis. Table 16-3 presents a small sampling of clinical information that can be ascertained from these techniques.

TABLE 16-3 ▶
Applications of Immunofluorescence

Clinical Laboratory Analyses
Identification of lymphocyte populations in blood
Detection of serum autoantibody in serum or tissue
Detection of tissue-fixed complement components
Rapid identification of microorganisms
Detection of tumor antigens
Detection of transplantation antigens
Location of specific hormones and enzymes
Identification of chromosome banding patterns

CELL-MEDIATED IMMUNITY

Cell Counting

In addition to evaluating humoral immunity, there are multiple methods of evaluating the cellular component of the immune system. Undoubtedly, one of the most useful of these methods is the complete blood count (CBC). The CBC provides information on the numbers of each type of leukocyte present in the blood. However, the CBC alone says little about the functional capacity of the cell types that were counted. Cell-counting studies can be extended to FACS analysis to count B and T lymphocytes. In addition, the numbers of CD4 and CD8 T cells can be evaluated. Again, these tests provide information on the numbers of cells in the circulation, but they do not provide information on how many of those cells are functional.

Cell Function

There are many methods available to evaluate the functioning of the cellular components of the immune system. Some of these methods depend on direct analyses of cell metabolism, while other methods are more indirect.

B-cell function is easily measured by evaluating serum antibody levels. If the serum antibody levels are normal and the patient is able to make an appropriate response to an administered antigen, then the B-cell component of the immune system is functional, and if there is the appropriate isotype switch, the CD4 Th2 component of the immune system is also active.

Karen, the patient in the clinical case, was evaluated for her response to yeast antigens by measuring her skin reaction to soluble antigens derived from the yeast *Candida albicans*. In this test, antigen is deposited intradermally. The antigen can be phagocytosed by the Langerhans' cells (local macrophages of the skin) and presented to the CD4 Th1 lymphocytes. Since Karen was recently infected with the organism, there should be a significant number of cells capable of reacting with the class II major histocompatibility complex (MHC II)–processed antigen complex. The response of CD4 Th1 cells should produce a significant amount of interferon-γ, resulting in a delayed-type hypersensitivity (DTH) response that is detected by evaluating the indurated swelling around the site of the antigen administration. The DTH skin test provides a method of evaluating CD4 Th1 cell function. Karen did not exhibit a significant response to the antigen, suggesting either that there was a problem with her T cells or that her previous yeast infections were not caused by *C. albicans*. To distinguish between the two possibilities, Karen's physician evaluated her response to a battery of common environmental antigens. Because Karen had been immunized to both mumps and measles, her physician included both of these antigens as positive skin test controls. All of her responses to the selected antigens were significantly lower than expected, suggesting that her immune system was somehow compromised, and that she was anergic.

In addition to in vivo DTH reactions, there are a number of methods available for evaluating lymphocyte responses in vitro. One method of stimulating lymphocytes in vitro is the mixed lymphocyte reaction. For this evaluation, lymphocytes from individuals expressing different MHC antigens are mixed in cell culture and allowed to respond to each other. The response can be measured by evaluating the release of cytokines from the activated cells, by measuring DNA synthesis, or by monitoring cell proliferation. An alternate method of stimulating lymphocyte proliferation is culturing the cells in the presence of mitogens and, again, evaluating cytokine production or following some other indicator of cell proliferation. Antigen-specific activation can be followed in a similar manner. These techniques are more commonly used in laboratories focused on clinical immunology research, since routine clinical laboratory tests and DTH skin testing, along with clinical data, provide a fairly comprehensive set of laboratory studies with which to evaluate the immune response.

> The differential component of the CBC provides percentages of the leukocyte populations. It is essential to convert these numbers to absolute cell counts. For example, a significant elevation in the total white blood cell (WBC) count may be associated with a decrease in the percentage of lymphocytes. This does not necessarily indicate a decrease in the number of lymphocytes, rather it may simply indicate an increase in the numbers of other cell types.

> The term anergy *can be defined in multiple ways, based on which test of the immune system is used to evaluate immunologic responses.* **Anergy** *indicates an absence of immune responses to antigens to which the host was previously sensitive or exposed.*

PHAGOCYTIC CELL FUNCTION

Although antibody-coated microorganisms can be cleared by cells of the reticuloendothelial system, antibody coating alone is usually insufficient to kill microorganisms. Effective antibody-dependent cell-mediated cytotoxicity (ADCC) depends upon auxillary cells and factors, such as the phagocytic cells and complement. An abnormality in either complement or phagocytes decreases the effective immune response to the organism.

Phagocytic cells must perform three functions in response to an antigen. The cell must be able to (1) detect the chemotactic factors liberated by the selected lymphocyte and migrate to the site of the inflammation, (2) phagocytose the opsonized antigen, and

(3) activate its lysosomal enzymes and oxidative mechanisms to kill the organism. There are diseases associated with abnormalities in each of these functions.

There are multiple methods to test each function. Phagocyte migration can be evaluated by observing the cell move to the source of a known chemotactic factor. Phagocytosis can be evaluated by culturing phagocytes with opsonized particles and then counting the number of phagocytosed particles per cell after a defined culture period. Enzyme or oxidative killing mechanisms can be evaluated directly by specific enzyme measurements or by chemically trapping the free radicals that are generated by activated phagocytes and measuring the reaction product. The nitroblue tetrazolium (NBT) reduction test is an example of this type of assessment of phagocyte function.

COMPLEMENT

Problems in the complement cascade can also lead to a successful bacterial infection, even in the presence of an appropriate antibody response. Tests of the complement system have been discussed in a previous chapter (see Chap. 14). The most direct approach is simply to determine complement activity using the CH50 evaluation. If complement function is missing, specific tests of the system are required to identify the missing component.

RESOLUTION OF CLINICAL CASE

Given Karen's age and history, her physician proceeded to evaluate her immune system in more detail. A detailed history identified a series of different infections over the past year; therefore, the first test that Karen's physician requested was an evaluation of antibody to the human immunodeficiency virus (HIV). The test indicated that Karen had been exposed and responded to HIV. Moreover, flow cytometric measurements using FACS showed that her T-cell levels were slightly lower than expected levels.

Karen was started on a course of antiviral chemotherapy. Throughout her continued treatment, the numbers of both her CD4 and CD8 lymphocytes were routinely determined to monitor her response to therapy.

REVIEW QUESTIONS

Directions: For each of the following questions, choose the **one best** answer.

1. Antibody concentrations in two different serum samples were compared by mixing 1 mL of each serum sample with a fixed concentration of antigen. Serum A resulted in a precipitate; serum B did not. Which of the following statements is a correct interpretation of these data?

   (A) Serum A contains antibody to the antigen, whereas serum B does not.

   (B) Both serum A and serum B contain antibody to the antigen.

   (C) Both serum A and serum B contain antibody to the antigen, but serum A contains more antibody than serum B.

   (D) Serum A contains antibody to the antigen. Conclusions about the antibody concentration in serum B or the relative concentrations of antibody in serum A and serum B are not possible.

2. Serum from an individual suffering from the sudden onset of symptoms of a cold was tested to evaluate the level of antibody to the specific influenza virus affecting the community. The results showed high levels of immunoglobulin G (IgG) antibody to the influenza virus. Which of the following is the correct interpretation of these data?

   (A) The individual is suffering from influenza.

   (B) This test cannot possibly be correct because the immune system uses cell-mediated immunity to respond to viral infections.

   (C) The individual is not sick.

   (D) The individual is not suffering from the current strain of the influenza virus but was exposed in the past.

3. Which of the following statements best describes the difference between agglutination reactions and precipitation reactions?

   (A) Precipitation reactions depend on the aggregation of antigen and antibody, whereas agglutination reactions only require antibody to bind a single antigen.

   (B) In agglutination reactions, either the antigen or antibody is insoluble, whereas in precipitation reactions both antibody and antigen are soluble until a complex is formed.

   (C) Agglutination reactions can only be used to measure bacteria.

   (D) Soluble antigens cannot be detected in agglutination reactions.

4. A patient presented with symptoms that suggested a bacterial infection. Serologic analyses of different bacterial strains revealed the following information: streptococcal antigen immunoglobulin G (IgG) titer = 2; streptococcal antigen IgM titer = 128; staphylococcal antigen IgG titer = 128; and staphylococcal antigen IgM titer = 2. Which of the following conclusions correctly interprets these data?

   (A) The patient, most probably, was suffering from a staphylococcal infection.

   (B) The patient, most probably, was suffering from a streptococcal infection.

   (C) The patient had suffered from a streptococcal infection in the recent past.

   (D) The data provide no information about the patient's previous exposure to disease.

5. A patient presented with the complaint of recurrent gastrointestinal (GI) disturbances. Analysis revealed that he had an elevated level of serum immunoglobulin A (IgA). The most likely explanation for this is which one of the following?

   (A) There is a major abnormality in the IgA system, because IgA is the antibody of the mucosal secretions.

   (B) There is a blood infection that specifically activates the IgA system.

   (C) The GI problems allow elevated levels of antigen to cross the intestinal barrier and stimulate the immune system.

   (D) There is no relationship between the finding of IgA antibody in the serum and the GI problems.

6. A patient with an acute onset of a streptococcal infection of the throat had a complete blood count (CBC) in which the white blood cell (WBC) count was significantly elevated. The differential showed that the percentage of neutrophils was also significantly elevated. All other cell populations were within normal limits except the lymphocytes, which were 15% of total cells (normal 20%–40%). These data are most consistent with which of the following statements?

   (A) The patient's infection is probably the result of an insufficient number of lymphocytes.

   (B) Lymphocytes do not play a role in antibody responses, so the decreased number of lymphocytes is not relevant to the infection.

   (C) The patient's lymphocyte count is probably normal.

   (D) The decreased lymphocyte count interferes with the generation of antibody immunity.

7. A patient had all of the expected symptoms of a tuberculosis infection. To confirm the suspected disease, while waiting for the results of the sputum culture, the physician evaluated the patient's delayed-type hypersensitivity reactions to several antigens. The results showed the following:

Antigen	Induration (mm) [Negative < 5 mm]
Purified protein derivative (PPD)	4 mm
Mumps	3 mm
Measles	3 mm

   The data are most consistent with which of the following statements?

   (A) The patient does not have a tuberculosis infection.

   (B) The patient's infection does not stimulate CD4 Th1 lymphocytes.

   (C) The patient may be anergic.

   (D) The patient has a human immunodeficiency virus (HIV) infection.

8. As part of a pre-employment physical, an individual was given a battery of delayed-type hypersensitivity skin tests with the following results:

Antigen	Induration (mm) [Negative > 5 mm]
Purified protein derivative (PPD)	13 mm
Mumps	15 mm
Measles	16 mm
Brucellosis	2 mm

   The results are most consistent with which of the following statements?

   (A) The patient is immune deficient and is suffering from multiple infections.

   (B) The patient has tuberculosis.

   (C) The patient is anergic.

   (D) The patient has been exposed to tuberculosis.

9. When reagent containing antibody to human immunoglobulin is mixed with a patient's erythrocytes, the cells agglutinate. This reaction is most likely caused by which of the following serum antibody populations?

   (A) Antibody to erythrocyte antigens in the patient's serum.

   (B) Antibody to the antihuman immunoglobulin reagent in the reagent.

   (C) The absence of antibody to erythrocyte antigens in the patient's serum.

   (D) The absence of antibody to the antihuman immunoglobulin reagent in the reagent.

10. A patient had a normal number of CD4 and CD8 cells in his blood but had been stricken with several viral infections that resolved very slowly and with difficulty. Which of the following immunologic conditions is most consistent with this finding?

    (A) The antibody titer to the virus infection is elevated.

    (B) The antibody titer to the virus infection is suppressed.

    (C) The number of T cells is insufficient to respond adequately to the virus infections.

    (D) T cells are present, but their function must be evaluated.

ANSWERS AND EXPLANATIONS

1. **The answer is D.** Because serum A reacted with the antigen, there is clearly antibody to the antigen or an antibody that cross-reacts with the antigen. Serum B, on the other hand, is unknown. Serum B could have no antibody present, or it could have such large concentrations of antibody that the resulting immune complexes were small and the ratio of antigen to antibody was in a zone of antibody excess.

2. **The answer is D.** The data indicate a previous exposure to the specific influenza virus. If the individual was currently suffering from the virus, the immune system would begin its humoral and cell-mediated responses to that agent. If antibody were detected, it would be expected to be of the IgM class.

3. **The answer is B.** The precipitation and agglutination reactions are similar in all respects, except that agglutination reactions imply that one component of the reaction mixture is insoluble. The insoluble particle may be a bacteria, an erythrocyte, a latex particle, or another insoluble matrix. Both precipitation reactions and agglutination reactions can be used to measure soluble antigens by evaluating the inhibition of precipitation or agglutination.

4. **The answer is B.** Whereas immunochemical data alone do not provide conclusive information that the symptoms were caused by a streptococcal organism, the IgM and IgG antibody levels indicate a very recent infection that has not as yet had the necessary time to switch antibody isotypes. The high IgG titer for the staphylococcal organism indicates that the patient was recently exposed and successfully responded to that organism.

5. **The answer is C.** All antibody isotypes can be measured in the serum. IgA antibody generated in the mucosal-associated tissues adds to the serum antibody concentration. When there is an increased response to mucosal antigens, representative antibody from that response can be detected in the blood.

6. **The answer is C.** In evaluating the differential cell percentages, it is essential to consider absolute cell numbers. An increase in total white blood cells associated with a decrease in the percentage of a cell population may indicate a normal number of cells.

7. **The answer is C.** The battery of antigens with which the patient was tested includes not only tuberculosis but also antigens to which the patient had most probably been immunized. These results are consistent with anergy. The reason for the lack of immunologic responses is not clear, given the data.

8. **The answer is D.** These data are consistent with a healthy immune system. Common antigens to which the individual has been exposed are positive, and antigens to which the patient has not been exposed are negative. The PPD response in the absence of a clinical indication of infection must be further evaluated. A positive PPD test could indicate disease, but it also might indicate previous immunization or exposure to the antigen.

9. **The answer is A.** This is an example of the Coombs' test. Human antibody on the erythrocyte membrane agglutinates in the presence of a second antibody.

10. **The answer is D.** In this situation cell numbers are normal, yet clinical information indicates that there is a problem with cell-mediated immunity. The most likely scenario is that there may be a functional problem with the lymphocytes, which must be evaluated.

17
IMMUNODEFICIENCY

INTRODUCTION OF CLINICAL CASE

Jake Osborn, a 4-year-old who had not been immunized, acquired a measles infection. Prior to his case of measles, he was a normal 4-year-old, having experienced many routine childhood infections. Jake's illness followed the predicted course for measles until he was ready to return to his normal routine. At that point, Jake experienced the sudden onset of a high temperature and vomiting. Moreover, Jake had periods of altered consciousness. Jake was rushed to the hospital, where he experienced a seizure. Jake's cerebrospinal fluid (CSF) analysis indicated a normal glucose level and a significantly elevated white blood cell (WBC) count. All of these data are consistent with a viral encephalitis infection secondary to the measles infection.

Jake experienced no unusual childhood illnesses other than the measles. However, this unexpected infection came on while he was recovering from the measles, suggesting that there may have been some abnormality or deficiency in Jake's immune system that put him at greater risk for acquiring a secondary infection.

Infection with the measles virus significantly increases the risk of acquiring encephalitis or any of several other secondary infections. In underdeveloped countries, secondary infections are a major cause of the morbidity and mortality associated with the virus.

Deficiencies of the immune system can be divided into two broad categories. Congenital deficiencies are genetic and are defined as primary immunodeficiencies. The second category includes deficiencies that indirectly result from some other event or condition. These are secondary, or acquired, immunodeficiencies.

PRIMARY IMMUNODEFICIENCY

Outlining the development of the immune system, each *arrow* in Fig. 17-1 represents multiple developmental steps. Developmental errors can occur in any of these steps. To complicate the problem further, errors vary in both magnitude and severity of conse-quence. These errors may include an absolute blockade of the pathway, preventing further development, an abnormal number of cells and factors, or an alteration in normal cell function in the presence of normal cell numbers. Consequently, the clinical presen-tation can vary considerably, and identifying specific lesions in different pathways can challenge the physician's problem-solving skills. However, with an understanding of the functions for each cell type and knowledge of cytokine activities and the infections experienced by the patient, it is possible to identify fairly accurately the site of a suspected developmental lesion in the immune system. Table 17-1 presents some possible effects on the immune system caused by lesions at the developmental steps shown in Fig. 17-1. Most of the immunodeficiencies in Table 17-1 are rare. The excep-tion is the selective deficiency of IgA antibody, which occurs in approximately 1 in every 700 individuals.

FIGURE 17-1 ▶

Development of the Immune System. Each of the numbers in this figure repre-sents a site where a developmental error in the immune system could occur. Each site may represent a total blockade in develop-ment, or it may represent a partial error. If the development of the stem cell popula-tion (site 1) failed, there would be a total reticular dysgenesis. Developmental errors in the nonlymphoid stem cells (site 2 or site 3) would compromise the functions of multiple cell populations, such as the erythrocytes, granulocytes, and mono-cytes. Examples of such developmental errors include aplastic anemia and phagocyte deficiencies, such as chronic granulomatous disease. A developmental error in the generation of the lymphoid stem cell (site 4) would compromise the function of both humoral and cellular immunity. A total failure at site 4 would result in a severe combined immune deficiency. A developmental problem may occur as the lymphoid stem cell differenti-ates either into the T-cell lineage (site 5) or into the B-cell lineage (site 7). If the prob-lem were in the development of T cells (DiGeorge syndrome) then one would ex-pect abnormalities in delayed-type hyper-sensitivity (DTH) and cytotoxic reactions. Moreover, one would expect the lack of an isotype switch and memory in the humoral immune response. If the problem were in the development of the B-cell lineage (congenital agammaglobulinemia), then the T-cell responses to viral antigen and DTH responses should be relatively intact, but one would expect difficulty in the re-sponse to bacteria. Developmental errors are also possible in the differentiation pro-cess as cells mature into the various types of T cells. Moreover, in the B-cell popula-tions, selective immunoglobulin (IgG, IgE, IgA) deficiencies are also observed.

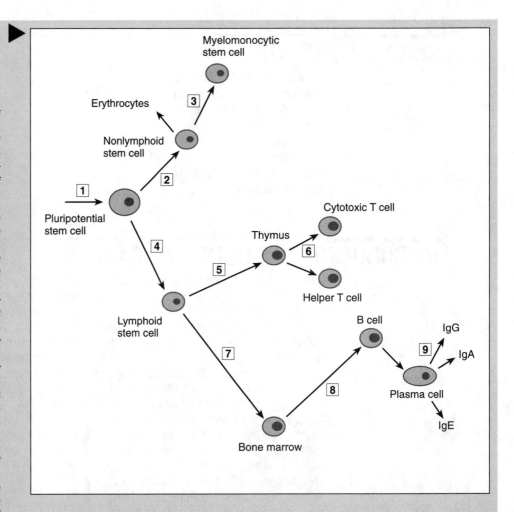

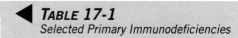

TABLE 17-1
Selected Primary Immunodeficiencies

Step Number[a]	Immunodeficiency	Effect on the Immune System
4	Severe combined	No B- or T-cell immunity
5	DiGeorge syndrome (thymic hypoplasia)	T-cell deficiency (serum IgM antibody present, but no isotype switch is possible)
7 and 8	Bruton's agamma-globulinemia	Deficient serum antibody, functional T-cell immunity
9	Selective isotype deficiency	Missing a selected antibody isotype

[a] See Fig. 17-1.

SECONDARY IMMUNODEFICIENCY

Far more common than most of the primary immunodeficiencies are the secondary, or acquired, immunodeficiencies. These are defined as a hypofunctioning of the immune system resulting from some other factor or event. Jake's immune system was compromised by his measles infection, so he was unable to mount successfully an immune response to the encephalitis virus. This is but one example of a secondary immunodeficiency. In measles infection, the highly infectious virus induces a massive immune response that is associated with leukopenia, a systemic secretion of cytokines, and increased glucocorticoid production. Together, these events produce a temporary immunosuppressed state. This transient immunodeficiency allows the establishment of secondary infections. In addition to the immune response itself inducing a transient immunosuppression, there are several common causes of acquired immunodeficiency.

Nutritional

Throughout the world, the most common form of immunodeficiency is that which is secondary to malnutrition. As expected, both the humoral and cell-mediated immune systems are affected by malnutrition, and the mechanism of the deficiency, although not well defined, relates to calorie, vitamin, and mineral limitations in leukocyte development.

Iatrogenic

Secondary immunodeficiency is also generated by medical treatment procedures. Both radiation therapy and antineoplastic agents clearly suppress the active proliferation required to mount successfully an immune response. Moreover, several therapeutic reagents have well-defined bone marrow toxicity, which can interfere with the continued production and development of leukocytes. These agents also can suppress red blood cell (RBC) production.

Infectious

Jake's secondary immunosuppression resulted from his immune response to an infectious agent. The immune system itself can be infected, which obviously can lead to altered immune responses. One well-known agent that can infect the immune system is the human immunodeficiency virus (HIV), which affected the patient in Chap. 16. The biology of and effect on the immune system of HIV is extensively covered in recent reviews and most current immunology textbooks. HIV, however, is only one of many organisms that can infect immunocompetent cells and alter their responsiveness. Human T-cell leukemia virus (HTLV-1) infects CD4 cells, activating instead of suppressing their responses, and Epstein-Barr virus (EBV) can infect B lymphocytes.

In addition to the organisms themselves that infect cells of the immune system, several bacteria and viruses have evolved protective mechanisms that actively suppress the immune responses. The mechanisms employed by these organisms are ingenious, encompassing mechanisms such as superantigen expression, which results in a massive release of cytokines that paralyze the immune system, as well as factors that interfere with major histocompatibility complex function and factors that alter phagocyte function. The numerous mechanisms employed by these organisms to escape the immune system are fascinating but go well beyond this introductory text.

RESOLUTION OF CLINICAL CASE

When Jake contracted measles, his immune system mounted an active response in all tissues. The virus infects many cells, including cells of the immune system, in which the massive cytokine production leads to leukopenia. Moreover, the stress responses associated with the infection, along with other normal immunoregulatory mechanisms, effectively suppress the immune system. Jake's transient immunocompromised state permitted colonization by other infectious agents. Secondary infections can involve colonization of any of the organ systems with either viruses or bacteria. In Jake's case, secondary infection resulted in encephalomyelitis.

REVIEW QUESTIONS

Directions: For each of the following questions, choose the **one best** answer.

1. A patient was seen for repeated viral and bacterial infections. Serum analyses showed elevated levels of the immunoglobulin M (IgM) antibody. Antibodies of the IgG, IgA, and IgE isotypes were missing. Which of the following is the most likely explanation for these data?

   (A) An error in the generation of the lymphoid stem cell
   (B) An error in the B-cell developmental pathway
   (C) An error in the T-cell developmental pathway
   (D) An error in phagocyte function

2. A patient experienced repeated bacterial infections. The infections were controlled only with aggressive antibiotic therapy and were associated with the formation of multiple granulomas. The serum antibody levels to several common bacteria were elevated. Which of the following is the most likely explanation for these data?

   (A) An error in the generation of the lymphoid stem cell
   (B) An error in the B-cell developmental pathway
   (C) An error in the T-cell developmental pathway
   (D) An error in phagocyte function

3. Which of the following conditions is best described as a primary immunodeficiency?

   (A) Failure of the immune system to develop properly because of a nutritional deficiency
   (B) Failure of the immune system to generate antigen-binding diversity because of lack of a critical enzyme
   (C) Immunodeficiency resulting from cancer chemotherapy
   (D) Immunodeficiency following human immunodeficiency virus (HIV) infection

4. Which of the following abnormalities is best described as a secondary immunodeficiency?

   (A) Selective deficiency of IgA antibody production
   (B) Failure of the T-cell population to mature, secondary to structural and functional alteration of the thymus gland
   (C) Immunodeficiency following radiation exposure
   (D) Failure to make the IgG, IgE, and IgA antibodies, secondary to the lack of helper T lymphocytes

5. Which of the following would be the most likely finding in a patient whose T lymphocytes failed to develop?

   (A) No antibodies are present in serum.
   (B) Analysis of serum antibodies reveals IgM only.
   (C) Analysis of serum antibodies reveals only IgM and IgA antibodies.
   (D) Analysis of serum antibodies reveals only IgG, IgE, and IgA antibodies.

ANSWERS AND EXPLANATIONS

1. **The answer is C.** The repeated viral infections point to a problem with the T-cell component of the immune system. The problem with the antibody deficiencies of the IgG, IgE, and IgA isotypes in the presence of IgM suggests a deficiency in helper T-cell function rather than a B-cell developmental problem.

2. **The answer is D.** Repeated bacterial infections suggest a problem with the humoral immune system. The chronic granuloma formation identifies the Th1 cells as functioning properly and compensating for the lack of humoral immunity. The elevated antibody levels suggest that the problem is not in the B-cell component of the immune system but rather in the methods of killing the antibody-coated cells. The two most obvious choices for the error, then, are either the complement system or the granulocytes.

3. **The answer is B.** Congenital deficiency of an enzyme such as adenosine deaminase interferes with proper DNA synthesis. This is a primary, or congenital, immunodeficiency. Adenosine deaminase deficiency causes severe combined immunodeficiency.

4. **The answer is C.** All of the other answer choices for this question describe a congenital problem. In choice C, a previously functional immune system was rendered nonfunctional by radiation exposure.

5. **The answer is B.** In a patient whose T cells fail to develop, the B-cell component of the immune system is functional, and B cells are able to respond to T-independent antigens with an IgM response. T-cell help for isotype switching, B-cell proliferation, and memory would be missing.

INDEX

Note: Page numbers in *italics* refer to illustrations; page numbers followed by t refer to tables.